NEUROBLASTOMA

A Guide for Parents,
Patients, and Families

Dr. Bhratri Bhushan MD, DM

Copyright © 2024 Dr. Bhratri Bhushan

Copyright © 2024 by Dr. Bhratri Bhushan

All rights reserved. No part of this publication may be reproduced, distributed, or transmitted in any form or by any means, including photocopying, recording, or other electronic or mechanical methods, without the prior written permission of the publisher, except in the case of brief quotations embodied in critical reviews and certain other noncommercial uses permitted by copyright law.

For permission requests, write to the publisher, addressed "Attention: Permissions Coordinator," at the address:

A30, Ananta institute of medical sciences,
Rajsamand, Rajasthan, India 313202
Email: www.bhratri@gmail.com

This work is provided "as is," and the author and the publisher disclaim any and all warranties, express or implied, including any warranties as to accuracy, comprehensiveness, or currency of the content of this work.

To the maximum extent permitted under applicable law, no responsibility is assumed by the publisher for any injury and/or damage to persons or property as a matter of products liability, negligence law or otherwise, or from any reference to or use by any person of this work.

CONTENTS

Title Page
Copyright
Preface
Introduction   1
Clinical Presentation   4
Workup for Suspected Neuroblastoma   7
Pathology   13
Imaging   20
Staging and Risk Classification   27
Treatment for Patients with non-high risk Neuroblastoma   30
Treatment for High-Risk Neuroblastoma   36
Response Assessment in Neuroblastoma   49
Disease Surveillance in Neuroblastoma   52
Monitoring for Late Effects of Neuroblastoma Treatment   60
Complications of Neuroblastoma Treatment   64

Principles of Treating Neuroblastoma: A Detailed Discussion	70
Pathology: An In-Depth Exploration	71
Surgery: An In-Depth Exploration	82
Systemic Therapy: An In-Depth Exploration	93
Radiation Therapy: An In-Depth Exploration	109
Primary Tumor Response Assessment: An In-Depth ExploratioN	112
A Letter to Families	118
About The Author	121

PREFACE

Neuroblastoma can be an overwhelming diagnosis, not just for the child but for their entire family. As parents, caregivers, or loved ones, navigating the complexities of this condition—its diagnosis, treatment, and potential outcomes—can feel like stepping into an unfamiliar and daunting world. The journey is filled with questions, decisions, and emotions, and at times, it may seem like there are more uncertainties than answers.

This book was born out of a heartfelt desire to provide clarity, comfort, and empowerment to those facing this challenging journey. Written with compassion and informed by years of medical expertise, "Neuroblastoma: A Guide for Parents, Patients, and Families" seeks to bridge the gap between medical knowledge and the lived experience of families affected by this disease.

Our aim is to demystify the science, explaining

complex medical concepts in clear, understandable language while offering practical insights into navigating the healthcare system and managing treatments.

Whether you are at the beginning of this journey, seeking to understand the basics, or looking for in-depth information about treatment options and long-term care, this guide is designed to meet you where you are. Every chapter has been thoughtfully written to provide knowledge and support while respecting the individual paths that each family and patient may take.

We hope this book becomes a trusted companion, answering your questions and alleviating your fears. More than that, we hope it reminds you that you are not alone in this fight and that there is a community of people—medical professionals, caregivers, survivors, and advocates—who are here to support you every step of the way.

INTRODUCTION

Neuroblastoma is a type of cancer that starts in the sympathetic nervous system, which is part of the body's nervous system that controls certain automatic functions like heart rate and digestion. It is the most common solid tumor found outside the brain in children. In the United States, over 700 new cases are diagnosed each year, and it is estimated to occur in about 1 out of every 7,000 live births. Most children diagnosed with neuroblastoma are very young, usually between 1 and 2 years old, with the majority being 4 years old or younger.

This cancer develops from immature nerve cells called neuroblasts, which are part of the neuroectodermal tissue. These tumors can appear anywhere in the body where the sympathoadrenal neuroendocrine system is present, such as the adrenal glands (located above the kidneys), soft tissues, the area behind the abdomen (retroperitoneum), and the chest (mediastinum).

Neuroblastoma is a highly variable disease, meaning its severity and behavior can differ widely from one person to another. In some cases, the tumor may disappear on its own without treatment, while in others, it may spread aggressively to other parts of the body, requiring intensive therapies like surgery, chemotherapy, and radiation. The complexity of neuroblastoma also means that symptoms and outcomes vary greatly depending on the specific characteristics of the tumor.

Beyond the challenges of the disease and its treatment, some families face additional hurdles due to disparities in healthcare. Studies suggest that outcomes, such as survival rates, can be influenced by factors like race, ethnicity, and socioeconomic status.

Genetic Risk Factors

Neuroblastoma develops due to genetic and molecular abnormalities that disrupt normal development of the sympathetic nervous system. While the exact cause of neuroblastoma is not fully understood, the following are the most accurate and well-documented contributing factors:

1. Sporadic Genetic Mutations:
   - The majority of neuroblastoma cases are sporadic, arising from somatic mutations in tumor cells. These mutations often occur in genes involved in cell growth and differentiation.

2. Familial Genetic Mutations (Rare, 1–2% of cases):
   - Inherited germline mutations in genes like ALK (anaplastic lymphoma kinase) and PHOX2B can predispose individuals to familial neuroblastoma.

3. Segmental Chromosomal Aberrations (SCAs):
   - Loss or gain of chromosomal material (e.g., 1p

deletion, 11q deletion, or 17q gain) can promote tumor development and progression.

4. MYCN Amplification:
   - Amplification of the MYCN oncogene is a critical driver in aggressive forms of neuroblastoma and is strongly associated with poor prognosis.

5. Abnormal Embryonic Development:
   - Neuroblastoma originates from neural crest cells, which are precursors of the sympathetic nervous system. Disruptions in the normal development or differentiation of these cells can lead to tumor formation.

6. Environmental and External Factors:
   - No specific environmental exposures have been definitively linked to neuroblastoma, and it is not typically associated with inherited syndromes outside of genetic predispositions.

These factors contribute to the complexity of neuroblastoma, which is influenced by a combination of genetic, molecular, and developmental abnormalities.

CLINICAL PRESENTATION

The symptoms of neuroblastoma vary depending on the tumor's location, size, and whether it has spread (metastasized). Common symptoms include:

General Symptoms

- Fatigue
- Loss of appetite
- Weight loss
- Fever
- Irritability

Localized Tumor Symptoms

1. Abdominal Tumor (most common site):
   - Abdominal swelling or mass (may feel firm and painless).
   - Abdominal pain.
   - Constipation or difficulty urinating due to compression of organs.

2. Chest Tumor:
   - Difficulty breathing.
   - Chest pain.
   - Compression of blood vessels, leading to swelling in the face, neck, or upper body.

3. Paraspinal Tumor:
   - Weakness or paralysis of the lower extremities (if the spinal cord is compressed).

- Back pain.

Metastatic Symptoms

1. Bone Pain:
   - Due to bone or bone marrow involvement.
2. Bruising or Swelling Around the Eyes:
   - Often called "raccoon eyes," caused by orbital bone metastases.
3. Anemia, Bleeding, or Infections:
   - From bone marrow infiltration.
4. Swollen Lymph Nodes:
   - Enlarged nodes may be felt in the neck, armpits, or groin.

Paraneoplastic Syndromes

Paraneoplastic syndromes are a group of rare disorders that arise as indirect effects of a malignancy, caused not by the direct invasion of cancer cells but by the immune system's response to the tumor or substances secreted by the tumor itself. These syndromes can affect various organ systems, including the nervous, endocrine, and hematologic systems, as well as the skin. They often manifest with symptoms that are disproportionate to the size or spread of the tumor, sometimes even preceding a cancer diagnosis. Paraneoplastic syndromes result from the production of hormones, cytokines, or antibodies by the tumor, which disrupt normal cellular function in distant parts of the body. Recognizing these syndromes is crucial, as they can provide an early clue to the presence of an underlying malignancy and significantly impact the management and prognosis of affected individuals.

- Opsoclonus-Myoclonus-Ataxia Syndrome (OMAS):
    - Rapid, jerky eye movements (opsoclonus).
    - Muscle jerks (myoclonus).
    - Coordination problems (ataxia).
    - Irritability and sleep disturbances.
- Hypertension:
    - Caused by catecholamine secretion by the tumor.

Symptoms of Specific Organ Involvement

- Liver Enlargement:
    - Common in infants with metastases.
- Skin Nodules:
    - Bluish lumps indicating metastatic spread to the skin.

When to Suspect Neuroblastoma

- A firm abdominal or chest mass.
- Unexplained symptoms such as bone pain, bruising, or fever.
- Paraneoplastic symptoms like OMAS or hypertension.

If neuroblastoma is suspected, medical evaluation with imaging, laboratory tests, and possible biopsy is essential for diagnosis.

WORKUP FOR SUSPECTED NEUROBLASTOMA

When neuroblastoma is suspected in a child outside the perinatal period (the time immediately before, during, and shortly after birth—typically from 22 weeks of gestation to 7 days postpartum), a thorough diagnostic process is required. This involves tissue sampling, a complete medical history, family history evaluation, laboratory tests, and imaging studies. Tissue evaluation is critical not only to confirm the diagnosis but also to classify the tumor's risk level and guide treatment decisions.

Diagnostic Criteria

To make a definitive diagnosis, one of the following criteria must be met:
1. Pathologic Diagnosis: Tumor tissue must show definitive neuroblastoma features under light microscopy.
2. Bone Marrow and Urinary Catecholamines: The presence of neuroblastoma cells in bone marrow aspirate or biopsy (e.g., tumor syncytia or clumps of immunocytologically positive cells) along with elevated levels of urinary catecholamine metabolites.

Tissue Sampling and Biopsy

- Surgical Resection vs. Biopsy:

- Surgical resection is considered in cases of localized disease without image-defined risk factors (IDRFs).

- If biopsy is required instead of resection, minimally invasive techniques (e.g., core biopsies) are preferred. However, an open biopsy may be necessary in cases where enough tissue cannot be obtained by less invasive means.

- Fine-Needle Aspiration (FNA): Not recommended, as it does not provide sufficient tissue for complete evaluation.

- Pathology Review: An experienced pathologist should review frozen sections of the tissue to ensure sample adequacy. Some samples may be necrotic and unsuitable for analysis.

What are IDRFs?

IDRFs are Image-Defined Risk Factors. These are specific features seen on imaging studies that indicate a higher risk of complications during surgical resection of a neuroblastoma tumor. These risk factors highlight tumor involvement with vital structures, such as major blood vessels, organs, or the spinal cord, and help guide treatment decisions by identifying patients who may require preoperative chemotherapy or alternative management strategies to reduce surgical risks. Recognizing IDRFs is an essential part of the International Neuroblastoma Risk Group Staging System (INRGSS).

For adequate diagnostic and prognostic evaluation, enough tissue must be collected for:
- Histologic evaluation to examine the cellular characteristics of the tumor.
- Molecular testing to assess key prognostic markers and support risk classification.

When possible, additional tissue should be preserved for research purposes, but this should only occur after clinical needs are met.

Special Considerations

1. Bone Marrow Biopsy: In rare cases where the bone marrow is the only source of tumor cells, bilateral bone marrow aspirates and biopsies can be used for diagnosis. Sufficient material for molecular testing should still be prioritized.

2. Infants and Young Children:
   - For patients under 2 months of age with rapidly enlarging livers (hepatomegaly) or those too unstable for biopsy (e.g., due to bleeding risks or organ failure), treatment may be initiated before biopsy, with tissue collection delayed until the patient is stable.
   - Infants under 6 months of age with small, localized adrenal tumors (≤3.1 cm solid or ≤5 cm if cystic) may not require an initial biopsy or resection. This approach is supported by research showing good outcomes in these low-risk cases.

The workup not only confirms the diagnosis but

also determines the tumor's stage and risk level, which are crucial for selecting the appropriate treatment plan. This tailored approach helps maximize the chances of successful outcomes while minimizing unnecessary treatments.

Additional Workup

A thorough and systematic approach for all patients suspected of having neuroblastoma is a must. This includes physical examinations, laboratory tests, and imaging studies, each contributing to diagnosis, staging, and treatment planning.

Physical Examination

A complete history and physical (H&P) is critical:
- Abdominal Exam: Focus on detecting masses or organ enlargement (organomegaly).
- Neurologic Exam: Assess for any signs of nervous system involvement, such as weakness or changes in reflexes.
- Family History: Record any instances of neuroblastoma or other childhood cancers, as familial cases, though rare, have implications for genetic counseling and management.

Laboratory Tests

Essential tests include:
1. Complete Blood Count (CBC) with Differential: To identify anemia, pancytopenia, or other blood abnormalities.

2. Comprehensive Metabolic Panel: To evaluate kidney and liver function and detect metabolic disturbances.

3. Urinary Catecholamine Levels (HVA and VMA):

- Elevated homovanillic acid (HVA) and vanillylmandelic acid (VMA) levels are seen in most neuroblastoma patients.

- These tests are crucial for diagnosis when bone marrow is the primary diagnostic tissue.

Additional laboratory tests for specific scenarios

- PT/INR: Recommended if the liver is involved or there are concerns about bleeding risks.
- Lactate Dehydrogenase (LDH) and Ferritin Levels: High levels of these markers can indicate a worse prognosis, but they are not part of the formal risk classification system.
- Pregnancy Test: Required for patients of childbearing potential to ensure safety during treatment.
- Fertility Referral: Patients with high-risk disease should consult fertility specialists to discuss options for fertility preservation.

Specialized Assessments

Some evaluations depend on the anticipated treatment:

- Audiograms: Recommended if ototoxic chemotherapy agents are planned.
- Echocardiograms or Electrocardiograms: Necessary if chemotherapy agents with potential

cardiac side effects are part of the treatment regimen.

PATHOLOGY

A coordinated diagnostic sampling and pathology workflow is crucial in diagnosing neuroblastoma and determining its risk classification. Collaboration among pathologists, oncologists, surgeons, and radiologists ensures that tissue samples meet the requirements for histologic diagnosis, prognostic classification, and molecular profiling.

Tissue Sampling for Neuroblastoma

- Tissue Collection Methods:
  - Surgical resection (if clinically indicated).
  - Incisional biopsy (sample size >1 cm^3).
  - Core needle biopsies (at least 10 cores, ideally 20–30 mm long, obtained with a 16-gauge needle).
- Special Considerations:
  - Bilateral bone marrow biopsies alone may not suffice for full risk assessment.
  - Open biopsies may be necessary when minimally invasive procedures cannot provide adequate tissue.
  - Tissue should be prepared in various formats (e.g., formalin-fixed paraffin-embedded [FFPE], fresh, frozen) to facilitate comprehensive testing.

For clinical trials, additional tissue testing may be

required, necessitating advanced planning during sampling. Fine-needle aspiration (FNA) is not recommended due to insufficient sample size for detailed evaluation.

Histologic Classification of Neuroblastoma

The International Neuroblastoma Pathology Classification (INPC) system is the gold standard for classifying neuroblastoma. Tumors are categorized based on:

1. Histologic Features:
   - Assessed through hematoxylin and eosin (H&E) staining.
2. Immunohistochemistry:
   - Markers such as chromogranin, synaptophysin, PHOX2B, and tyrosine hydroxylase are useful for confirming neuroblastoma in small or unusual samples.

Neuroblastoma belongs to a group of tumors derived from the sympathetic nervous system. The INPC classifies these tumors into four categories based on the presence of Schwannian stroma:

1. Neuroblastoma (Schwannian stroma-poor).
2. Ganglioneuroblastoma, Intermixed (Schwannian stroma-rich).
3. Ganglioneuroma (Schwannian stroma-dominant).
4. Ganglioneuroblastoma, Nodular (a composite

of stroma-rich/stroma-dominant and stroma-poor regions).

Among these, neuroblastoma is the most common. Tumors such as ganglioneuroblastoma (intermixed) and ganglioneuroma are generally found in older children, classified as Favorable Histology, and associated with excellent prognoses.

Favorable vs. Unfavorable Histology

Tumors are classified based on three factors:
1. Neuroblastic Differentiation:
   - Undifferentiated, poorly differentiated, or differentiating subtypes.
2. Mitosis-Karyorrhexis Index (MKI):
   - Reflects the number of dividing and dying cells per 5,000 tumor cells:
     - Low (<100), Intermediate (100–200), High (≥200).
3. Age at Diagnosis:
   - Younger patients generally have better outcomes.

- Favorable Histology:
  - Includes younger patients (<548 days or <1824 days for specific subtypes) with low to intermediate MKI and differentiating or poorly differentiated tumors.
- Unfavorable Histology:
  - Includes older patients, tumors with

undifferentiated subtypes, or high MKI at any age.

For ganglioneuroblastoma, nodular, the prognosis depends on the neuroblastoma component, and the same criteria as neuroblastoma are applied.

Key Prognostic Insights
- Favorable histology tumors, such as ganglioneuroblastoma (intermixed) and ganglioneuroma, have excellent outcomes.
- Neuroblastoma tumors with unfavorable histology require more intensive treatment due to poorer prognoses.

This structured approach to pathology ensures accurate diagnosis and prognostic stratification, forming the basis for individualized treatment planning.

Molecular Genetic Testing

Molecular genetic testing is a cornerstone for determining the risk classification and initial treatment plan for neuroblastoma. Key prognostic biomarkers include MYCN amplification, segmental chromosomal aberrations (SCAs), and tumor cell ploidy. These factors help stratify patients into risk groups and guide therapy.

Key Molecular Biomarkers

1. MYCN Amplification:
   - Amplification of the MYCN oncogene is

the strongest independent prognostic marker in neuroblastoma.

- It is associated with aggressive disease and poor outcomes.

- Assessment of MYCN status is recommended for all neuroblastomas, including nodules in ganglioneuroblastoma nodular tumors.

2. Segmental Chromosomal Aberrations (SCAs):

- SCAs involve gains or losses of portions of chromosome arms and are linked to poorer prognoses.

- The most commonly studied SCAs in neuroblastoma include:

  - Losses: Chromosomes 1p, 11q, 3p, 4p.
  - Gains: Chromosomes 17q, 1q, 2p.

- Testing for these seven SCAs is recommended to ensure accurate risk stratification.

3. Ploidy Status:

- Reflects the amount of DNA in tumor cells and is expressed as the DNA index (DI).

- DI = 1 (diploid) is less favorable compared to DI >1 (hyperdiploid).

- Ploidy is particularly important for risk classification in infants.

Emerging Molecular Targets

- New targeted therapies are being developed for neuroblastoma. For instance, genetic alterations in the ALK gene (amplifications or mutations) can predict responsiveness to specific targeted

treatments.
- As therapies evolve, testing protocols will adapt to include additional biomarkers.

Testing Techniques and Assay Selection

1. Next-Generation Sequencing (NGS):
   - NGS is widely available and feasible for analyzing formalin-fixed paraffin-embedded (FFPE) tissue.
   - It allows simultaneous evaluation of:
     - MYCN amplification.
     - SCAs.
     - Other actionable genetic alterations, such as ALK mutations.
   - NGS is particularly advantageous when tissue samples are limited, as it enables comprehensive assessment in a single assay.

2. Fluorescence In Situ Hybridization (FISH), Microarray, and Flow Cytometry:
   - These methods can detect MYCN amplification, copy number changes, and SCAs.
   - However, they cannot identify sequence variants in neuroblastoma-related genes, such as mutations in ALK.

Practical Considerations

- A single, robust assay (e.g., NGS) is often preferable when tissue is limited to ensure all relevant biomarkers are assessed efficiently.

- Testing should be planned carefully to capture essential prognostic markers while conserving tissue for potential future analyses or research.

As the landscape of neuroblastoma treatment evolves, molecular genetic testing will continue to play an essential role, offering insights into both prognostic risk and therapeutic opportunities.

IMAGING

Imaging plays a critical role in diagnosing, staging, and managing neuroblastoma. The choice of imaging studies depends on the patient's symptoms, tumor location, and the suspected extent of disease. It helps confirm the diagnosis, assess local tumor extension and metastatic spread, plan surgery, and evaluate treatment response.

Goals of Imaging

1. Identify imaging features consistent with a neuroblastic tumor.
2. Assess for Image-Defined Risk Factors (IDRFs) to aid in staging and evaluate surgical risks.
3. Determine the extent of regional and distant metastases.
4. Facilitate post-treatment response evaluation and long-term disease surveillance.

The choice of imaging studies for initial evaluation depends on the patient's symptoms and suspected sites of disease involvement. Neuroblastoma frequently exhibits local extension, which may include vascular encasement, infiltration into nearby soft tissues and organs (commonly the kidneys and liver), or invasion of the foramina and epidural space when the tumor originates from the paraspinal sympathetic chain. About 50% of patients present with localized or regional disease, and 35% have lymph node involvement at diagnosis.

The International Neuroblastoma Risk Group (INRG) Task Force developed the INRG Staging System (INRGSS) and the accompanying risk classification system to guide imaging and treatment planning. Radiology plays an increasingly vital role in these systems. Unlike the earlier approach of measuring tumor volume, the revised International Neuroblastoma Response Criteria (INRC) uses RECIST (Response Evaluation Criteria in Solid Tumors) to measure the longest dimension of soft tissue disease.

The primary goals of imaging are to confirm features consistent with a neuroblastic tumor, identify image-defined risk factors (IDRFs) for staging (L1 or L2), assess the potential surgical risks, evaluate the presence and extent of regional and distant metastases, and aid in response assessment and disease monitoring after treatment.

Ultrasound (US) is often the first imaging modality used when an abdominal or pelvic tumor is suspected in a child. It is noninvasive, widely available, and avoids radiation exposure. However, its utility is limited by low interobserver consistency and challenges in evaluating calcified tumors due to acoustic shadowing. While ultrasound is useful for initial screening, magnetic resonance imaging (MRI) or computed tomography

(CT) is necessary for accurate staging and treatment planning.

CT and MRI are both essential for evaluating soft-tissue disease. CT is preferred for its rapid availability, superior detection of calcifications, and reduced need for sedation due to fast image acquisition. In contrast, MRI is better suited for assessing spinal involvement and avoids ionizing radiation. Both modalities are often used during the initial evaluation, particularly for paraspinal tumors, and are effective in detecting primary tumors and metastases in the liver, lymph nodes, bone, and skin. Together, these imaging techniques provide critical information for staging, surgical planning, and ongoing disease monitoring.

IDFRs

Imaging is a cornerstone of the diagnostic workup and plays a significant role in tumor staging and risk classification. Image-Defined Risk Factors (IDRFs) are critical imaging features that indicate an increased risk of surgical complications due to tumor location and its relationship to nearby vital structures. Recognizing IDRFs helps determine the complexity of surgical resection and guides treatment planning. The following are descriptions of IDRFs categorized by anatomic region:

1. Multiple Body Compartments
- Tumor extends within two adjacent body

compartments, such as:
- Neck and chest.
- Chest and abdomen.
- Abdomen and pelvis.

2. Neck
- Tumor encases:
  - Carotid artery, vertebral artery, and/or internal jugular vein.
- Tumor extends to the skull base.
- Tumor compresses the trachea.

3. Cervicothoracic Junction
- Tumor encases:
  - Brachial plexus roots.
  - Subclavian vessels, vertebral artery, and/or carotid artery.
- Tumor compresses the trachea.

4. Thorax
- Tumor encases:
  - Aorta and/or its major branches.
- Tumor compresses the trachea and/or principal bronchi.
- Lower mediastinal tumor infiltrates the costovertebral junction at T9–T12 vertebral levels.

5. Abdomen and Pelvis
- Tumor infiltrates the porta hepatis and/or hepatoduodenal ligament.
- Tumor encases:
  - Branches of the superior mesenteric artery at the mesenteric root.

- Origin of the celiac axis and/or superior mesenteric artery.
  - One or both renal pedicles.
  - The aorta and/or vena cava.
  - Iliac vessels.
- Pelvic tumor crosses the sciatic notch.

6. Intraspinal Tumor Extension
- Tumor occupies more than one-third of the spinal canal in the axial plane.
- Perimedullary leptomeningeal spaces are not visible.
- Spinal cord shows abnormal signal intensity.

7. Infiltration of Adjacent Organs and Structures
- Tumor infiltrates the:
  - Pericardium.
  - Diaphragm.
  - Kidney.
  - Liver.
  - Duodenopancreatic block.
  - Mesentery.

8. Thoracoabdominal Junction
- Tumor encases the aorta and/or vena cava.

These IDRFs help classify tumors as L1 or L2 under the INRG Staging System and are instrumental in assessing surgical risks, guiding preoperative therapy, and determining the optimal timing and approach for tumor resection.

Nuclear Imaging in

Neuroblastic Tumors

Nuclear imaging plays a crucial role in the evaluation and management of neuroblastic tumors, particularly for identifying metastatic disease. The most commonly used agent is Iodine-123 metaiodobenzylguanidine (123I-MIBG), which is highly specific and sensitive for detecting neuroblastoma tumors due to its uptake by norepinephrine transporters. This characteristic allows MIBG imaging to localize metastatic sites with exceptional accuracy, making it the preferred diagnostic imaging tool in neuroblastoma. MIBG uptake is demonstrated in approximately 90% of neuroblastoma tumors, underscoring its utility in the diagnostic process.

Timing and Indications:

123I-MIBG imaging is recommended prior to the surgical resection of the primary tumor whenever possible. However, it may not be required in specific scenarios, such as in infants younger than 6 months with localized adrenal tumors of ≤3.1 cm in diameter if solid or ≤5 cm if the tumor contains at least 25% cystic components. Baseline MIBG imaging can also be delayed in patients younger than 2 months or those weighing less than 2.5 kg who have suspected primary adrenal tumors. While novel radiotracers are under development, they are not yet widely adopted due to insufficient data.

Technical Considerations:

In addition to whole-body planar scintigraphy (covering the vertex of the head to the feet), SPECT or SPECT/CT imaging is recommended for sites of known or suspected disease, where available, as these techniques improve sensitivity and anatomic localization. MIBG imaging is interpreted using semiquantitative scoring systems, such as the modified Curie score (commonly used in North America) and the SIOPEN score (used in Europe). These systems allow for a standardized evaluation of tumor uptake across body segments.

Alternative Imaging Modalities:

When neuroblastoma tumors are not MIBG avid or when there is a discrepancy between MIBG findings and anatomic imaging, FDG-PET/CT or PET/MRI serve as valuable supplemental or alternative diagnostic tools. Additionally, Iodine-131 MIBG (131I-MIBG), while less commonly used, may be a viable option in resource-limited settings.

MIBG imaging is essential for accurately identifying the extent of disease, particularly metastatic spread, and for guiding treatment decisions in neuroblastoma patients. It remains the gold standard in nuclear imaging for this condition, with FDG-PET/CT providing support in cases where MIBG imaging is insufficient.

STAGING AND RISK CLASSIFICATION

Staging and risk classification are essential in neuroblastoma as they guide treatment strategies and predict outcomes. The International Neuroblastoma Risk Group Staging System (INRGSS) and the Children's Oncology Group (COG) risk classification system are widely used to ensure consistent and effective management.

Staging with INRGSS

The INRGSS stages neuroblastoma based on imaging and clinical findings before the initiation of treatment. This system categorizes tumors into stages L1, L2, M, and MS, incorporating Image-Defined Risk Factors (IDRFs).

1. Stage L1:
   - Localized tumor confined to one body compartment.
   - No IDRFs present (e.g., no involvement of vital structures).

2. Stage L2:
   - Locoregional tumor with one or more IDRFs.
   - IDRFs indicate potential challenges in surgical removal and may reflect tumor biology.

3. Stage M:
   - Distant metastatic disease.

- Commonly involves bone marrow, bones, liver, or lymph nodes.

4. Stage MS:
   - Diagnosed in children <18 months of age.
   - Metastases are limited to the skin, liver, and/or bone marrow (with minimal marrow involvement).

Risk Classification

The COG risk classification system incorporates factors such as age, stage, MYCN amplification, histopathology, chromosomal aberrations (SCAs), and ploidy to assign patients to low-risk, intermediate-risk, or high-risk groups.

1. Low-Risk Group:
   - L1 tumors without MYCN amplification.
   - L1 tumors with MYCN amplification, but only if completely resected.
   - MS tumors in asymptomatic infants <12 months, with:
      - Favorable histology.
      - MYCN non-amplified.
      - Hyperdiploid.
      - Absence of SCAs.

2. High-Risk Group:
   - L1 tumors with residual MYCN-amplified disease post-resection.
   - M or MS stage disease in patients ≥12 months with:
      - Unfavorable histology.

- SCAs or MYCN amplification.
 - All patients ≥18 months with M stage disease.
 - Detection of MYCN amplification in any age or stage (except fully resected L1 disease).

3. Intermediate-Risk Group:
 - Patients who do not meet the criteria for low- or high-risk categories.
 - Includes symptomatic MS infants where a biopsy is deferred due to critical illness (e.g., respiratory compromise from hepatomegaly). These patients may be reassigned to the high-risk group if later biopsy shows MYCN amplification.

Special Considerations

- International Differences: The COG risk classification differs from those used outside North America. For example, L2 tumors in patients >18 months with unfavorable histology or undifferentiated/poorly differentiated tumors are high risk in the COG system but may be intermediate risk elsewhere.
- Emergent Therapy: If urgent treatment is needed (e.g., respiratory compromise or coagulopathy), imaging and biopsy may be deferred temporarily. Risk classification must be revisited after stabilization and completion of testing.

TREATMENT FOR PATIENTS WITH NON-HIGH RISK NEUROBLASTOMA

The treatment of neuroblastoma is highly individualized, requiring the expertise of a multidisciplinary team that includes radiologists, pathologists, surgeons, oncologists, and nuclear medicine specialists. Treatment strategies depend on the disease's risk classification, with distinct approaches for non–high-risk and high-risk neuroblastoma.

Non–High-Risk Disease

Approximately half of all newly diagnosed neuroblastoma patients fall into the non–high-risk category, which includes low-risk and intermediate-risk groups. These patients generally have excellent survival rates:
- Low-Risk Disease: >95% five-year survival.
- Intermediate-Risk Disease: 90%–95% five-year survival.

Treatment Goals

The primary objective for non–high-risk patients is to cure the disease while minimizing treatment-related toxicity. Recent advances in therapy have focused on reducing treatment intensity for patients with favorable biology, achieving excellent outcomes while lowering the burden of treatment.

Treatment for Low-Risk Neuroblastoma

1. Surgical Resection:
  - For patients with INRG L1 tumors (localized without IDRFs), surgical removal is typically the primary treatment.
  - Surgery aims to:
    - Cure the disease.
    - Avoid the need for chemotherapy if the tumor is fully resected.
  - If the tumor cannot be fully resected:
    - Patients with MYCN amplification are reclassified as high-risk.
    - Further treatment decisions are based on tumor biology and patient characteristics.

2. Observation:
  - Infants (<6 months) with isolated adrenal tumors:
    Observation without biopsy is recommended if:
    - The tumor is ≤3.1 cm in diameter (solid).
    - The tumor is ≤5 cm if at least 25% cystic.
  - INRG MS disease with favorable biology:
    - Asymptomatic patients are best managed with observation.

3. Chemotherapy:
  - Reserved for rare cases where the tumor causes complications or cannot be managed by surgery or

observation alone.
- The goal is to use the minimum effective dose to control the disease.

Key Principles

- Treatment decisions are guided by tumor biology and clinical presentation.
- Favorable biological features (e.g., absence of MYCN amplification, hyperdiploidy, absence of SCAs) often allow for less intensive treatment.
- Observation is increasingly favored in specific scenarios to avoid unnecessary interventions.

Treatment for Intermediate-Risk Neuroblastoma

Treatment for intermediate-risk neuroblastoma typically involves a combination of moderate-intensity chemotherapy and surgical resection. The aim is to balance disease control with minimizing toxicity, preserving organ function, and achieving acceptable outcomes for this group of patients, who generally have a five-year survival rate of 90%–95%.

Key Principles of Treatment

1. Chemotherapy:
   - Patients receive 2 to 8 cycles of chemotherapy.
   - The number of cycles depends on:
     - Disease stage.
     - Tumor biology (e.g., histology, ploidy, and chromosomal aberrations).

- Age at diagnosis.
- Favorable tumor biology features include:
  - Favorable Histology.
  - DNA Index (DI) > 1.
  - Absence of SCAs.
- When biologic features (e.g., SCA or histology) are unavailable, clinicians should assume unfavorable features for treatment planning.
- Commonly used chemotherapy agents include cyclophosphamide and topotecan.

2. Surgical Resection:
- Surgery is used to achieve tumor reduction when chemotherapy alone does not meet the response targets.
- Timing and feasibility are assessed based on:
  - The tumor's response to chemotherapy.
  - Risks to vital structures and organ function.
- A resection is appropriate if chemotherapy results in <50% tumor reduction, but the preservation of vital structures is paramount.

3. Response Goals:
- The primary treatment endpoint is achieving sufficient tumor reduction:
  - ≥50% reduction for tumors with favorable biology.
  - ≥90% reduction (very good partial response, VGPR) for tumors with less favorable biology.
- Response is measured using either:
  - Tumor volume (legacy criteria).
  - Single longest dimension (RECIST criteria).

4. Observation and Surveillance:
- After achieving the targeted tumor reduction, patients enter a surveillance phase without additional treatment.
- If targets are not met, the treatment team must discuss further chemotherapy cycles, surgery, or alternative strategies.

Special Scenarios

1. Unstable Patients:
- Infants with stage MS disease who cannot undergo biopsy (e.g., due to organ failure or coagulopathy) are started on chemotherapy with biopsy deferred until stabilization.

2. Residual Tumor:
- For tumors that do not sufficiently shrink:
- A biopsy of the residual mass can help determine whether the tumor has differentiated histologically, potentially supporting observation.
- If surgery is unsafe, additional chemotherapy may be administered, followed by reevaluation every 2 cycles.

3. Chemoresistant Tumors:
- For tumors that do not respond to the standard 8-cycle regimen:
- Cyclophosphamide and topotecan can be considered as salvage therapy.
- Similar treatment approaches from SIOPEN (European trials) may also be used, as outcomes are

comparable to COG strategies.

4. Multidisciplinary Discussions:
   - Decisions about timing, type, and intensity of additional treatments should involve surgeons, oncologists, radiologists, and pathologists to ensure a patient-centered approach.

Key Considerations

- The focus is on minimizing long-term complications while achieving disease control.
- Less than complete tumor response is often acceptable if it does not compromise survival, especially for localized intermediate-risk tumors.
- Risks and benefits of additional treatment steps (e.g., chemotherapy or surgery) should be reassessed iteratively based on disease response.

TREATMENT FOR HIGH-RISK NEUROBLASTOMA

High-risk neuroblastoma constitutes about half of newly diagnosed cases and poses significant challenges due to its aggressive nature. Despite advances in treatment, the estimated 5-year event-free survival (EFS) rate is approximately 51%, according to data from the Children's Oncology Group (COG). Management involves intensive multimodal therapy, divided into induction, consolidation, and post-consolidation phases.

Induction Therapy

The goal of induction therapy is to reduce tumor burden and achieve the best possible response prior to consolidation therapy.

Key Components:
1. Chemotherapy:
   - Multiagent regimens form the backbone of induction therapy.
   - Preferred regimens include:
     - ANBL12P1: Five-cycle induction regimen with proven efficacy and acceptable toxicity.
     - ANBL1531: A slightly modified version of ANBL12P1 aligned with updated COG standards.
     - ANBL0532: Six-cycle regimen, also acceptable.
   - Regimens typically include cisplatin, alkylators,

topotecan, and cyclophosphamide.

- End-induction response rates of 80% (partial response or better) are achieved with these regimens.

2. Stem Cell Collection:

- Autologous peripheral blood stem cells are harvested during induction for use in subsequent consolidation therapy.

3. Surgical Resection:

- Surgery to remove the primary tumor and locoregional disease is performed after several chemotherapy cycles.

- The goal is gross total resection (>90% of the tumor or macroscopic resection).

- Subtotal resection is acceptable when achieving gross total resection would compromise vital structures such as major blood vessels, nerves, or organs.

4. Response Assessment:

- Full disease reassessment is conducted at the end of induction.

- Patients achieving a partial response or better proceed to consolidation therapy.

- Patients with progressive disease are treated with non-myeloablative therapies or enrolled in clinical trials.

Management of Poor End-Induction Response

1. Progressive Disease:

- Patients with disease progression during or after induction are not candidates for standard consolidation therapy.
- Recommended strategies:
- Chemoimmunotherapy: Combining anti-GD2 monoclonal antibodies with chemotherapy.
- Participation in clinical trials.

2. Minor Response or Stable Disease:
   - Individualized decision-making is required.
   - Options include:
   - Bridging Therapy: Alternative therapies to improve response before proceeding to consolidation.
   - Consolidation Therapy: May be considered for patients whose disease improves significantly with bridging therapy.

Future Directions in Induction

- ALK Inhibitors: Early addition of ALK inhibitors for tumors with ALK aberrations is under investigation.
- Experimental Therapies:
  - 131I-MIBG therapy: Radioisotope-based targeted therapy.
  - Anti-GD2 monoclonal antibodies: To enhance immune-mediated tumor destruction.
  - These approaches are not yet standard but are available in clinical trials.

Outcomes and Considerations

- End-Induction Response:

- Patients with partial or better responses fare better in subsequent phases.
- Those with inadequate responses may benefit from bridging therapies or alternative regimens before consolidation.
- Consolidation Therapy:
  - Tandem transplant (two autologous stem cell transplants) has shown superior outcomes over a single transplant in trials like ANBL0532.
- Clinical Trials:
  - Enrollment in trials is encouraged to explore newer, potentially more effective strategies for high-risk neuroblastoma.

Consolidation Therapy

Consolidation therapy aims to further reduce disease burden following induction therapy and increase long-term survival. This phase typically includes high-dose chemotherapy with autologous stem cell rescue (HSCR) and radiotherapy.

Components of Consolidation Therapy

1. High-Dose Chemotherapy with Autologous Stem Cell Rescue

This approach has been a cornerstone of high-risk neuroblastoma treatment and is supported by data demonstrating improved outcomes compared to continued conventional chemotherapy.

- Tandem Transplantation:
  - Recommended for most patients with high-risk

disease (Category 1 recommendation).
- Based on the COG ANBL0532 trial, which demonstrated superior 3-year event-free survival (EFS) for tandem transplant (61.6%) compared to single transplant (48.4%).
- Tandem transplantation involves:
 - First transplant with thiotepa/cyclophosphamide.
 - Second transplant (6–10 weeks later) with dose-reduced carboplatin/etoposide/melphalan (CEM).

- Single Transplant:
- Recommended for specific subgroups with historically better outcomes:
 1. Stage L2:
  - Age ≥18 months, Unfavorable Histology, and MYCN non-amplified.
 2. Stage M:
  - Age 12 to <18 months, MYCN non-amplified, with unfavorable features (e.g., Unfavorable Histology, diploid DNA content, and/or SCAs).
- Single transplant with full-dose CEM is endorsed for these patients based on COG data showing 5-year EFS rates of 75%–80%.

- European Approach (BuMel Regimen):
- In Europe, busulfan/melphalan (BuMel) is preferred due to superior EFS compared to CEM in the rapid COJEC induction regimen.
- BuMel is associated with lower toxicity but an increased risk of sinusoidal obstruction syndrome.
- While BuMel has been piloted in North America,

its role in U.S. regimens is not yet established.

2. Radiation Therapy (RT)

Radiotherapy is administered after recovery from high-dose chemotherapy and stem cell rescue, targeting:

- Primary tumor site:
  - Standard dose: 21.6 Gy.
  - Augmented doses (e.g., additional 14.4 Gy for residual tumor) have not shown added benefit and are not recommended.
- Residual metastatic disease:
  - Sites identified via 123I-MIBG or FDG-PET (for MIBG non-avid disease) are targeted.
  - Not all metastatic sites may be feasibly treated with external beam radiotherapy (EBRT).
- Expanding RT fields to include uninvolved nodal stations has not improved outcomes and is not recommended.

Considerations for Consolidation Therapy

1. Emerging Evidence and Alternatives:
   - In the era of anti-GD2 immunotherapy, retrospective data suggest that patients with a partial response or better might achieve comparable outcomes with or without high-dose chemotherapy and HSCR. This finding warrants further investigation but is not yet standard practice.

2. Contraindications to Tandem Transplant:
   - Single transplant with BuMel or CEM may be appropriate for patients who cannot tolerate

tandem transplantation.

3. Radiotherapy Considerations:
   - Neuroblastoma is highly radiosensitive, but RT should balance efficacy with minimizing long-term side effects.
   - Decisions on RT for metastatic sites require careful planning, as not all sites may be accessible or safely treated.

Post-Consolidation Therapy for High-Risk Neuroblastoma

Post-consolidation therapy is critical in maintaining disease control and improving outcomes for patients with high-risk neuroblastoma after consolidation therapy. Anti-GD2 antibody-based therapy is recommended for patients without disease progression following consolidation, while chemoimmunotherapy or clinical trial participation is advised for those with progressive disease.

Standard Post-Consolidation Therapy

1. Anti-GD2 Monoclonal Antibody Therapy with Isotretinoin:
   - Based on the ANBL0032 trial, the combination of the anti-GD2 monoclonal antibody dinutuximab, cytokines (sargramostim and interleukin-2), and isotretinoin significantly improved event-free survival (EFS):
     - 2-year EFS with this regimen: 66%.
     - 2-year EFS with isotretinoin alone: 46%.

- This led to a Category 1 recommendation for anti-GD2 antibody therapy with isotretinoin.

2. Revised Protocols Without Interleukin-2:

- The SIOPEN HR-NBL1 trial demonstrated no benefit from adding interleukin-2 (IL-2) to anti-GD2 immunotherapy and associated IL-2 with increased toxicity.
- Current protocols in North America exclude IL-2 endorse anti-GD2 immunotherapy without IL-2.

3. Alternative Anti-GD2 Regimens:

- In Europe, dinutuximab beta combined with isotretinoin, without sargramostim or IL-2, is commonly used.
- Non-randomized comparisons show improved outcomes with this regimen compared to isotretinoin alone, supporting its use as an alternative post-consolidation therapy.

Role of Isotretinoin (Differentiating Agent)

- Isotretinoin remains a core component of post-consolidation therapy due to its established role in improving survival, as shown in the CCG-3891 trial.
- It is typically administered for 6 cycles to induce tumor cell differentiation and reduce the risk of relapse.

Special Considerations

1. Progressive Disease:

- Patients who progress during consolidation therapy are typically ineligible for standard post-

consolidation regimens.
  - Recommended options include:
    - Chemoimmunotherapy (e.g., combining anti-GD2 antibodies with chemotherapy).
    - Participation in clinical trials for innovative therapies.

2. Alternative Anti-GD2 Antibodies:
  - Other anti-GD2 antibodies (e.g., dinutuximab beta) may be used, especially in regions or scenarios where dinutuximab is not available.

Continuation Therapy for High-Risk Neuroblastoma

Eflornithine (DFMO), an inhibitor of ornithine decarboxylase, has emerged as a novel agent for continuation therapy in patients with high-risk neuroblastoma who achieve a partial response or better following frontline therapy. Its approval by the FDA in December 2023 underscores its growing role in improving outcomes for these patients.

Eflornithine in Continuation Therapy

1. Mechanism of Action:
  - Eflornithine inhibits ornithine decarboxylase, an enzyme critical for the synthesis of polyamines that support cancer cell survival and homeostasis.

2. Clinical Trial Evidence (Study 3b):
  - Phase 2 trial (NCT02395666) included children with high-risk neuroblastoma who responded

to induction, consolidation, and anti-GD2 immunotherapy.

- Patients received eflornithine (750 mg/m $\pm$ 250 mg/m² twice daily) for up to 2 years.

- Compared with an external control group treated with anti-GD2 immunotherapy and isotretinoin (from ANBL0032), eflornithine significantly improved outcomes:

   - Event-Free Survival (EFS): HR = 0.48 (95% CI, 0.27–0.85).

   - Overall Survival (OS): HR = 0.32 (95% CI, 0.15–0.70).

- Reported adverse events included transaminitis and hearing loss.

3. FDA Approval:

- Eflornithine is now approved as continuation therapy for patients with high-risk neuroblastoma who achieve at least a partial response post-immunotherapy.

- The guidelines suggest discussing eflornithine with patients and families.

4. Monitoring:

- Hearing evaluations (e.g., audiograms, brainstem auditory evoked responses) are crucial due to potential ototoxicity, especially in young children at critical ages for language development.

Disease Evaluation During Frontline Therapy

1. Key Timepoints:
   - Pre-Surgical Evaluation: Anatomic imaging (CT/MRI) of the primary site prior to surgery.
   - End of Induction: Full disease evaluation, including:
     - Anatomic imaging of the primary site.
     - 123I-MIBG scan (or FDG-PET for MIBG non-avid disease).
     - Bilateral bone marrow aspirates and biopsies.
   - Start of Post-Consolidation: Comprehensive disease assessment.
   - End of Therapy: Final disease evaluation to confirm response.

2. Residual Disease:
   - Patients with >5 MIBG-avid metastatic sites after induction should have a repeat 123I-MIBG scan post-consolidation to prioritize metastatic sites for radiotherapy.

3. Mid-Therapy Evaluations:
   - 123I-MIBG scans during post-consolidation therapy.
   - Bone marrow evaluations and anatomic imaging for patients with residual disease.

Organ Function Monitoring During Therapy

The intensive nature of high-risk therapy necessitates frequent and detailed monitoring of organ function to manage acute and long-term toxicities.

1. Renal Function:
   - Evaluated with glomerular filtration rate (GFR), often measured using nuclear medicine techniques, especially prior to high-dose chemotherapy.

2. Cardiac Function:
   - Regular echocardiograms and electrocardiograms are critical due to the cardiotoxicity risk of certain chemotherapeutic agents.

3. Hearing:
   - Audiograms or brainstem auditory evoked responses are essential to detect ototoxicity, particularly in young children.

4. Routine Laboratory Tests:
   - Frequent monitoring of blood counts, chemistry panels, and urinalysis is needed to manage therapy-related toxicity.

Considerations for Adolescents and Adults

While neuroblastoma predominantly affects young children, older patients occasionally present with high-risk disease. Key considerations include:

1. Treatment Principles:
   - The general principles of high-risk neuroblastoma therapy apply, but older patients may require more individualized approaches due to

comorbidities and potential therapy intolerance.

2. Limited Data:
   - Most clinical trials and toxicity data focus on patients <5 years of age, necessitating careful extrapolation of findings to older populations.

RESPONSE ASSESSMENT IN NEUROBLASTOMA

The guidelines recommend response criteria based on the International Neuroblastoma Response Criteria (INRC) revised in 2017. These updated criteria incorporate modern imaging techniques and improved methods for assessing bone marrow involvement, reflecting advances in neuroblastoma diagnosis and monitoring.

Key Components of Response Assessment

1. Primary Tumor and Metastatic Sites
   - Response is evaluated using:
     - RECIST (Response Evaluation Criteria in Solid Tumors) for measurable lesions.
     - Functional Imaging:
       - 123I-MIBG scans for MIBG-avid disease.
       - FDG-PET imaging for MIBG non-avid disease or when MIBG and anatomic imaging results do not align.
     - 123I-MIBG Uptake Scoring:
       - Assessed using semiquantitative systems:
         - Modified Curie Score (North America).
         - SIOPEN Score (Europe).
   - Technetium-99m (99mTc) bone scintigraphy is no longer recommended due to lower sensitivity and specificity compared to MIBG scans.

2. Bone Marrow Response
   - Bone marrow disease is evaluated using:
     - Immunocytology or immunohistochemistry, as described by Burchill et al in the INRC.
   - This approach ensures accurate detection of minimal residual disease (MRD) in the marrow.

3. Overall Response
   - Defined as the combined response across:
     - Primary tumor.
     - Metastatic bone and soft tissue lesions.
     - Bone marrow involvement.

Key Updates and Recommendations

1. Elimination of Urinary Catecholamines:
   - Changes in urinary homovanillic acid (HVA) and vanillylmandelic acid (VMA) levels are no longer used in response assessment due to:
     - Lack of standardization.
     - Influence of dietary factors.

2. Preferred Imaging Modalities:
   - MIBG Imaging:
     - High sensitivity and specificity for neuroblastoma.
   - Recommended for monitoring metastatic bone and soft tissue response.
   - FDG-PET:
     - Used for non-MIBG avid tumors or when discrepancies exist between MIBG and anatomic imaging.

- Novel radiotracers are under investigation but are not yet incorporated into routine practice due to insufficient data.

3. Response Timing:

- Timing of response assessments varies by risk group and phase of treatment. Clinicians should refer to specific algorithms for details.

DISEASE SURVEILLANCE IN NEUROBLASTOMA

Close surveillance is critical for detecting disease progression, relapse, or side effects from prior treatments. Surveillance strategies vary by risk group, ensuring tailored follow-up that balances vigilance with minimizing unnecessary interventions.

Surveillance for Low-Risk Neuroblastoma

A. Observation-Only Cases
- Ultrasound is the primary imaging modality for surveillance.
- Performed as clinically indicated, particularly for patients who did not require surgery or other therapies.

B. Post-Surgical Cases
1. Initial Cross-Sectional Imaging:
   - A baseline imaging study (e.g., CT or MRI) is recommended 1 month postoperatively to establish the new baseline after tumor resection.

2. Subsequent Surveillance:
   - Transition to ultrasound for routine follow-up, if feasible:
     - Every 3 months during the first year.

- Every 6 to 12 months during years 2–3.
- As clinically indicated thereafter.
- Cross-sectional imaging (e.g., CT or MRI) may still be required for surveillance in cases where the primary tumor location or other clinical factors warrant more detailed imaging.

3. Physical Exams:
 - Regular history and physical (H&P) exams are recommended:
    - Every 3 months during the first year.
    - Every 6 months during the second year.
    - Every 6 to 12 months during the third year.
    - As clinically indicated in subsequent years.

4. Laboratory Testing:
 - Urine Catecholamine Levels:
   - Not included in the revised INRC but may be considered during surveillance for patients who had elevated levels at diagnosis.
   - Testing should focus on spot catecholamine testing if clinically indicated.

Key Considerations for Low-Risk Disease

- Surveillance intensity is reduced over time, transitioning to less frequent imaging and clinical evaluations as the risk of relapse decreases.
- Decisions regarding imaging modality (ultrasound vs. cross-sectional imaging) should consider the tumor's initial location and the feasibility of detecting recurrence with ultrasound.

General Recommendations for Surveillance

For all risk groups, follow-up schedules and modalities are adapted to the patient's disease characteristics, treatment history, and clinical status. The aim is to ensure early detection of recurrence while avoiding unnecessary interventions that could increase patient burden or exposure to radiation.

Surveillance for Intermediate-Risk Neuroblastoma

Surveillance for patients with intermediate-risk neuroblastoma aims to monitor for disease recurrence or late treatment effects. Recommendations are derived from clinical trials (ANBL0531 and ANBL1232).

Surveillance Schedule

1. History and Physical Exam (H&P):
   - Every 3 months during year 1.
   - Every 6 months during year 2.
   - Annually during years 3–5.

2. Imaging:
   - End-of-Therapy Evaluation:
     - 123I-MIBG scan with SPECT (if available) for MIBG-avid tumors.
     - FDG-PET scan for MIBG non-avid tumors.
     - Imaging is repeated every 3–6 months in year

1, annually in years 2–3, and as clinically indicated, until a negative scan is achieved or the patient is 36 months post-therapy.
   - Primary Tumor Site Imaging:
     - CT or MRI:
       - Every 3 months during year 1.
       - Every 6 months during year 2.
       - Annually during year 3, then as clinically indicated.

3. Laboratory Testing:
   - Complete Blood Count (CBC) with Differential:
     - Recommended at the same frequency as imaging if bone marrow was involved at diagnosis.
   - Creatinine:
     - Every 6 months during year 1.
     - Annually during years 2–3.
     - As clinically indicated thereafter.
   - Thyroid Function (TSH and Free T4):
     - Annually for the first 3 years, then as clinically indicated.
   - Urine Catecholamine Levels:
     - No longer standard per the revised INRC but may be measured if elevated at diagnosis.

4. Audiologic Assessment:
   - Considered for patients exposed to ototoxic agents, such as platinum-based chemotherapies (e.g., cisplatin).

Key Considerations

1. MIBG or FDG-PET Imaging:

- If imaging at diagnosis and post-therapy is positive, scans should continue at defined intervals until a negative scan is achieved or 36 months post-therapy.

2. Late Effects Monitoring:
   - Thyroid dysfunction, renal impairment, and hearing loss are potential late effects of neuroblastoma therapy.
   - Surveillance protocols include targeted tests to detect and address these complications early.

3. Risk-Based Adjustments:
   - Surveillance intensity and specific tests may be modified based on the patient's clinical history, response to therapy, and risk of late effects.

Surveillance for High-Risk Neuroblastoma

Patients treated for high-risk neuroblastoma require long-term surveillance to monitor for relapse, late treatment effects, and complications associated with intensive therapy. Surveillance recommendations are adapted from the ANBL0532 and ANBL1531 studies.

Surveillance Schedule

1. History and Physical Exam (H&P):
   - Every 3 months during year 1.
   - Every 6 months during years 2–5.

2. Imaging:
   - 123I-MIBG Scan with SPECT:
     - Recommended for MIBG-avid tumors.
     - Every 3–6 months during year 1, every 6 months in year 2, then annually in year 3, and as clinically indicated.
   - FDG-PET:
     - Recommended for MIBG non-avid tumors.
   - Primary Tumor Site Imaging (CT or MRI):
     - Every 3–6 months during year 1.
     - Every 6 months in year 2.
     - Annually in year 3, then as clinically indicated.
   - Bone Marrow Evaluations:
     - If bone marrow involvement resolves by the end of therapy, further aspirates and biopsies are only performed if clinically indicated.

3. Laboratory Testing:
   - Complete Blood Count (CBC) with Differential:
     - Performed at the same frequency as imaging.
   - Electrolytes, Creatinine, ALT, and Bilirubin:
     - Every 3 months in year 1.
     - Every 6 months in years 2–3.
     - Annually in years 4–5.
   - Thyroid Function (TSH and Free T4):
     - Every 6 months in years 1–2.
     - Annually in years 3–5.
   - Urine Catecholamine Levels:
     - No longer recommended as part of routine surveillance but can be obtained if levels were elevated at diagnosis.

4. Audiologic Assessments:
   - Annually for 5 years due to the high prevalence of ototoxicity, especially in survivors exposed to cisplatin or other ototoxic agents.
   - Further evaluations as clinically indicated.

5. Cardiac Monitoring:
   - If cardiac function is normal at the end of therapy:
     - Obtain an echocardiogram every 2–5 years depending on cumulative anthracycline dose and radiation exposure.

6. Additional Evaluations:
   - Conduct the following as clinically indicated:
   - Hemoglobin A1c and ferritin (to monitor for late effects like metabolic syndrome or iron overload).
   - Reproductive Health Tests:
     - Follicle-stimulating hormone (FSH), luteinizing hormone (LH), anti-Müllerian hormone (AMH) for fertility assessment.
   - Pulmonary Function Tests if lung function was affected during therapy.

Key Considerations

1. Late Effects of Treatment:
   - Surveillance targets late toxicities associated with high-risk therapy, including:
     - Cardiotoxicity (anthracyclines, radiation).
     - Hearing loss (cisplatin).

- Thyroid dysfunction.
- Fertility issues and metabolic abnormalities.

2. Tailored Surveillance:
   - Adjust frequency and modalities based on:
   - Disease characteristics (e.g., MIBG avidity).
   - Treatment exposure (e.g., cumulative doses of nephrotoxic, ototoxic, or cardiotoxic agents).

3. Bone Marrow Evaluations:
   - Reserved for clinical indications if bone marrow was cleared by the end of therapy.

MONITORING FOR LATE EFFECTS OF NEUROBLASTOMA TREATMENT

The therapies used to treat neuroblastoma, particularly for high-risk disease, can lead to significant late effects that manifest months or years after treatment. Monitoring for these late effects is crucial for optimizing long-term outcomes and quality of life in survivors. A personalized survivorship care plan is essential, tailored to the patient's specific treatment history and individual risk factors.

General Monitoring Guidelines

- Monitoring for late effects typically begins 2 or more years after the completion of systemic therapy.
- Surveillance should be conducted at each follow-up visit and should evolve as the patient grows and matures.
- Survivors of high-risk neuroblastoma face the highest risk of long-term complications due to the intensity of treatments such as myeloablative therapy, radiotherapy, and high-dose chemotherapy.

Common Late Effects and Monitoring Recommendations

1. Hearing Impairment:

- Risk Factors: Platinum-based chemotherapy (e.g., cisplatin), eflornithine (13% risk of worsening hearing loss).

- Impact: Delays in speech/language development, academic performance, and social interactions.

- Monitoring:
  - Audiologic assessments per COG Survivorship Guidelines.
  - Referral to institutional audiology or otolaryngology teams for individualized follow-up schedules.

2. Endocrine Deficiencies:
- Risk Factors: Radiation to the head, neck, or spine; chemotherapeutic agents.
- Manifestations: Growth retardation, hypothyroidism, adrenal insufficiency, and pubertal delays.
- Monitoring:
  - Annual thyroid function tests (TSH, free T4).
  - Growth monitoring with height and weight charts.
  - Hormonal evaluations as clinically indicated.

3. Chronic Kidney Disease:
- Risk Factors: Nephrotoxic chemotherapies (e.g., cisplatin, ifosfamide) and radiotherapy.
- Monitoring:
  - Creatinine and GFR assessments at follow-up visits.
  - Annual renal function tests for patients with significant cumulative exposure.

4. Fertility Impairment:
   - Risk Factors: High-dose chemotherapy, radiation to the pelvic region.
   - Monitoring and Preservation:
   - Referral to fertility specialists before initiation of chemotherapy for discussion of fertility preservation options.
   - Long-term reproductive health monitoring.

5. Cardiotoxicity:
   - Risk Factors: Anthracycline-based chemotherapy (e.g., doxorubicin), radiation exposure.
   - Monitoring:
   - Echocardiograms and electrocardiograms (frequency depends on cumulative dose and radiation exposure).

6. Neurocognitive Impairment:
   - Risk Factors: Central nervous system toxicity from treatments.
   - Monitoring:
   - Neurocognitive evaluations if school performance or social skills are affected.

7. Second Malignant Neoplasms (SMNs):
   - Risk Factors: Radiation and certain chemotherapeutic agents.
   - Monitoring:
   - Regular screenings for thyroid and kidney cancers, as these are more common in survivors.
   - Adherence to COG Survivorship Guidelines for

secondary cancer risk.

Specific Recommendations by Risk Group

1. High-Risk Disease:
 - High rates of late morbidity, including endocrine, renal, and cardiac issues.
 - More intensive and frequent monitoring, especially for hearing, thyroid function, and secondary malignancies.

2. Intermediate- and Low-Risk Disease:
 - Generally lower risk of late effects due to reduced therapy intensity.
 - Heterogeneous treatment exposures warrant tailored follow-up based on individual therapy history.

Fertility Considerations

- Pre-Treatment Fertility Discussions:
 - Essential for patients with high-risk disease to explore fertility preservation options such as cryopreservation of gametes.
- Post-Treatment Monitoring:
 - Assessment of reproductive hormone levels (FSH, LH, AMH) as patients approach adolescence and adulthood.

COMPLICATIONS OF NEUROBLASTOMA TREATMENT

Treating neuroblastoma, particularly in high-risk cases, involves intensive therapies that, while effective in combating the disease, can lead to a wide range of acute and long-term complications. These challenges stem from the aggressive nature of the treatments, which include surgery, chemotherapy, radiation therapy, immunotherapy, and stem cell transplantation. Understanding these potential side effects allows families and caregivers to better prepare for and support the child during and after treatment.

Acute Complications

Acute complications arise during or shortly after treatment and depend on the specific therapies employed.

1. Complications from Surgery:

Surgery to remove tumors is often a critical part of neuroblastoma treatment. However, it carries risks such as infections at the surgical site, delayed wound healing, and bleeding. Depending on the tumor's location, surgery may inadvertently damage nearby organs or nerves, leading to complications like reduced mobility or chronic pain. Managing these risks involves careful surgical planning and postoperative care.

2. Complications from Chemotherapy:

Chemotherapy, a cornerstone of neuroblastoma treatment, works by targeting rapidly dividing cells, but it also affects healthy tissues. Common side effects include nausea, vomiting, and loss of appetite, often leading to weight loss. Hair loss is another frequent issue, though temporary. Blood cell counts are also affected, causing:

- Anemia (leading to fatigue and weakness).
- Neutropenia (making the child more prone to infections).
- Thrombocytopenia (increasing the risk of bruising and bleeding).

Additionally, chemotherapy can damage vital organs like the liver, kidneys, or heart, requiring close monitoring.

3. Complications from Radiation Therapy:

Radiation therapy, while highly targeted, can irritate the skin, causing burns or redness. Fatigue is another common side effect, as is the risk of damage to healthy tissues near the radiation site, depending on the tumor's location.

4. Complications from Immunotherapy:

Treatments like anti-GD2 antibodies are highly effective in targeting neuroblastoma cells but can cause significant pain during infusions. Other side effects include allergic reactions, fever, chills, and, in some cases, a drop in blood pressure. These effects are often managed with supportive medications and close monitoring.

5. Complications from Stem Cell Transplantation:

Stem cell transplants, used in high-risk cases, can lead to severe infections during the recovery period due to weakened immunity. In allogeneic transplants, graft-versus-host disease (GVHD) may occur, where the donor cells attack the recipient's body. Organ dysfunction, particularly of the liver and lungs, is another potential complication.

Long-Term Complications (Late Effects)

Late effects are complications that emerge months or years after treatment and can significantly impact a survivor's quality of life.

1. Hearing Loss:

Platinum-based chemotherapy drugs, such as cisplatin, and treatments like eflornithine can cause permanent hearing damage. Hearing loss may affect language development, academic performance, and social interactions, especially in young children.

2. Endocrine Problems:

Treatments involving radiation to the brain or spine and certain chemotherapies can disrupt hormone production, leading to growth delays, hypothyroidism, adrenal insufficiency, delayed puberty, or infertility. Lifelong monitoring of endocrine function is often necessary.

3. Cardiac Toxicity:

Anthracycline-based chemotherapies (e.g., doxorubicin) can damage the heart muscle, increasing the risk of heart failure or other cardiac issues later in life.

4. Kidney Disease:

Nephrotoxic agents and radiation therapy can lead to chronic kidney disease, which may require regular monitoring and interventions to manage.

5. Neurocognitive Impairment:

Children treated for neuroblastoma may experience difficulties with learning, memory, and attention due to the neurotoxic effects of treatments.

6. Psychosocial Challenges:

Survivors may face anxiety, depression, or difficulty reintegrating into school and social activities. Emotional and psychological support is often essential for both the child and their family.

7. Second Malignant Neoplasms (SMNs):

Radiation and certain chemotherapy agents increase the risk of developing secondary cancers, particularly in the thyroid or kidneys.

How Family Members Can Support the Child

Families play a central role in a child's treatment and

recovery, providing both practical and emotional support. Here's how families can help:

1. Emotional Support:

Be a source of reassurance and comfort. Validate the child's fears and feelings, and celebrate small victories to keep morale high. Patience is crucial, as mood swings or behavioral changes are common due to stress or treatment effects.

2. Medical Management:

- Stay organized by keeping track of medical appointments, medications, and follow-up tests.
- Watch for side effects or signs of complications, and promptly report them to the healthcare team.

3. Physical Health Promotion:

- Encourage a balanced diet rich in nutrients to support recovery and manage side effects.
- Help the child engage in gentle physical activities to maintain strength and mobility, as tolerated.
- Maintain strict hygiene practices to reduce the risk of infections.

4. Psychosocial Support:

- Create a sense of normalcy with routines like schoolwork and playtime.
- Join support groups for families of children with cancer to share experiences and seek advice.
- Seek professional counseling for emotional challenges.

5. Long-Term Care:

- Educate yourself about the potential late effects of treatment and stay vigilant for early warning signs.

- Ensure regular follow-ups and adherence to survivorship care plans.

- Advocate for the child's needs in school or other settings to ensure proper accommodations.

6. Self-Care for Caregivers:

- Take time to care for your own mental and physical health. This will ensure you can continue to provide the best support for your child.

PRINCIPLES OF TREATING NEUROBLASTOMA: A DETAILED DISCUSSION

The following chapters delve into the intricate details of the principles and approaches to treating neuroblastoma. It is designed for readers who wish to explore the technical aspects and gain a deeper understanding of the topic. However, if you prefer to skip the complexities and confine only to the practical or less detailed sections, feel free to do so. The content the previous chapters will still make sense and provide valuable insights without requiring prior knowledge of the technical details presented here.

PATHOLOGY: AN IN-DEPTH EXPLORATION

Key Principles

1. Workflow Design:
   - Pathology workflows must support histologic diagnosis, prognostic classification, and molecular profiling essential for treatment.

2. Tissue Requirements:
   - Evaluations:
     - Guided by clinical criteria for risk stratification and treatment selection.
     - Clinical trials may demand additional testing.
   - Tissue Considerations:
     - Primary Diagnosis (Tumor or Metastasis):
       - Surgical Resection: Performed if clinically indicated.
       - Incisional Biopsy: Requires specimens >1 cm^3.
       - Tissue Cores: Minimum of 10 cores; optimal length of 20–30 mm using a 16-gauge needle.
     - Bone Marrow Biopsies:
       - Bilateral biopsies and clot sections alone are insufficient for International Neuroblastoma Pathology Classification (INPC) requirements.

3. Challenges in Tissue Procurement:
   - Sufficient specimen quantity may necessitate

open surgical procedures over minimally invasive methods.

4. Specimen Handling:
   - Determine tissue condition requirements (e.g., FFPE, fresh, frozen, touch preparations) in advance to ensure all tests can be performed.

5. Team Coordination:
   - Diagnostic sampling benefits from collaboration between pathologists, oncologists, surgeons, and radiologists.

Histologic Classification (Neuroblastoma)

Diagnostic Standards
1. Reporting Guidelines:
   - Diagnosis follows ICCR (International Collaboration on Cancer Reporting) and INPC (International Neuroblastoma Pathology Classification).

2. Pre-Therapy Diagnosis:
   - INPC assessment must use diagnostic samples obtained before starting therapy.

3. Histologic Techniques:
   - Diagnosis primarily based on Hematoxylin and Eosin (H&E) staining.
   - In cases of small samples, unusual locations, or undifferentiated subtypes, immunohistochemical stains are useful:

- Neuronal Markers: Chromogranin, Synaptophysin.
- Neural Crest Marker: PHOX2B (strongly recommended), Tyrosine Hydroxylase.

Histopathological Findings in Neuroblastoma

Neuroblastoma, a malignant embryonal tumor of the sympathetic nervous system, typically arises from neural crest cells. It most commonly affects children under 5 years old. The histopathological evaluation of neuroblastoma plays a crucial role in diagnosis, prognostication, and treatment planning.

Key Histological Features

1. Tumor Composition
- Neuroblasts: The tumor is composed of small, round, blue neuroblastic cells. These cells have:
  - Hyperchromatic nuclei.
  - Scant cytoplasm.
  - High nuclear-to-cytoplasmic ratio.
- Neuropil: The hallmark of neuroblastoma is the presence of a fibrillary eosinophilic stroma, termed neuropil, which is composed of neuritic processes.

2. Differentiation Status
Based on the degree of differentiation, neuroblastoma can be classified into:
- Undifferentiated: Sheets of neuroblasts without neuropil or differentiation.
- Poorly Differentiated: Neuroblasts with some

neuropil and the presence of differentiating neuroblasts showing features like:
- Eccentric nuclei.
- Eosinophilic cytoplasm.
- Formation of rosettes (Homer Wright rosettes).
- Differentiating: A significant proportion of the tumor cells show ganglionic differentiation.

3. Homer Wright Rosettes
- Definition: Circular arrangements of neuroblasts around a central core of neuropil.
- Significance: These rosettes indicate neuronal differentiation but are not specific to neuroblastoma (also seen in other small round blue cell tumors).

4. Mitotic and Karyorrhectic Index (MKI)
- The MKI is a measure of mitotic and apoptotic activity.
- Classified into:
  - Low (<100/5000 cells).
  - Intermediate (100–200/5000 cells).
  - High (>200/5000 cells).
- A higher MKI is associated with a worse prognosis.

5. Stroma
- Neuroblastoma can be classified based on the amount of stroma:
  - Stroma-poor neuroblastoma: Mostly neuroblastic cells with little or no Schwannian stroma.
  - Stroma-rich neuroblastoma: Schwannian stroma predominates, associated with ganglioneuroblastoma or ganglioneuroma.

6. Calcification
- Psammoma body-like calcifications are often seen, especially in older tumors.

7. Vascularity and Necrosis
- The tumor is often highly vascular with areas of necrosis and hemorrhage, particularly in aggressive cases.

Histological Variants

1. Ganglioneuroblastoma:
   - Mixture of neuroblasts and ganglion cells.
   - Stroma-rich.
   - Better prognosis compared to pure neuroblastoma.

2. Ganglioneuroma:
   - Fully differentiated, benign form.
   - Composed entirely of ganglion cells and Schwannian stroma.

3. Schwannian Stroma-rich/Stroma-dominant Neuroblastoma:
   - Contains a mix of differentiated ganglion cells and Schwannian stroma.

Immunohistochemistry (IHC) Markers

1. Neuron-specific markers:
   - Synaptophysin and Chromogranin A: Indicate neuronal differentiation.
   - NSE (Neuron-Specific Enolase): Positive in

neuroblasts but less specific.
2. Proliferation marker:
   - Ki-67/MIB-1: High proliferation index indicates aggressive tumor behavior.
3. Schwannian markers:
   - S-100 protein: Positive in Schwannian stroma.
4. Other markers:
   - PHOX2B: A specific marker for neuroblasts.
   - CD56: Neural cell adhesion molecule often expressed.

Histopathological Prognostic Factors

1. Age:
   - Younger age (especially <18 months) is associated with better outcomes.
2. Differentiation:
   - Well-differentiated tumors have a better prognosis.
3. MKI:
   - Low MKI correlates with favorable outcomes.
4. Histological subtype:
   - Favorable (e.g., ganglioneuroma) vs. unfavorable histology (e.g., undifferentiated neuroblastoma).

INPC Prognostic Groups

1. Classification:
   - Favorable Histology (FH).
   - Unfavorable Histology (UH).

2. Tumor Categorization:
   - Schwannian Stroma-Poor (Neuroblastoma):
     - Subtypes:
       - Undifferentiated: Ancillary tests (immunohistochemistry/molecular analysis) critical.
       - Poorly Differentiated.
       - Differentiating Subtype.
   - Schwannian Stroma-Rich:
     - Ganglioneuroblastoma, Intermixed:
       - Biopsy diagnosis should note: "Favorable histology based on limited material," as sampling may miss neuroblastoma nodules.
     - Ganglioneuroma.
   - Composite Tumors:
     - Ganglioneuroblastoma, Nodular:
       - Contains stroma-rich/stroma-dominant and stroma-poor components.
       - Neuroblastoma component graded on degree of differentiation (undifferentiated, poorly differentiated, or differentiating).

Additional Parameters

1. Mitosis and Karyorrhexis Index (MKI):
   - Estimation of mitotic/karyorrhectic nuclei per 5000 neuroblastic cells.
   - Classifications:
     - Low MKI: <100/5000 cells.
     - Intermediate MKI: 100–200/5000 cells.
     - High MKI: ≥200/5000 cells.

2. Age at Diagnosis:
 - Plays a role in determining prognostic grouping.

Molecular Genetic Testing in Neuroblastoma

Prognostic Testing

1. Risk Stratification:
 - Molecular tumor profiling is crucial for primary treatment planning (refer to Principles of Risk Classification [NEUROB-C]).

2. MYCN Amplification:
 - Strongly associated with aggressive disease.
 - Testing is mandatory for:
   - All neuroblastomas.
   - Neuroblastomatous nodules of ganglioneuroblastoma nodular tumors.
 - Testing Methods:
   - Fluorescence In Situ Hybridization (FISH):
     - Not Amplified: 2 copies/cell.
     - Gain: >2–8 copies/cell or <4-fold increase.
     - Amplified: >8 copies/cell or ≥4-fold increase (up to >30-fold).
   - Microarray or Next-Generation Sequencing (NGS).

3. Segmental Chromosomal Aberrations (SCAs):
 - May correlate with aggressive disease, depending on other factors.

- Commonly studied SCAs:
  - 1p, 11q, 17q, 3p, 4p, 1q, 2p.
- Testing Methods:
  - Microarray or NGS.

4. Ploidy:
   - Measures DNA content in tumor cells.
   - DNA Index of 1:
     - May indicate aggressive disease, depending on age and other factors.
   - Testing Methods:
     - Flow Cytometry.
     - NGS (estimation).

Identification of Molecular Targets for Therapy

1. Targeted Therapy:
   - Emerging role in pediatric solid tumors, including neuroblastoma.
   - ALK Amplification/Sequence Variants:
     - Predict response to targeted agents.
   - Additional biomarkers may be tested as research and drug discovery progress.

Assay Selection for Molecular Testing in Neuroblastoma

Next-Generation Sequencing (NGS)
1. Advancements and Feasibility:
   - Widely available and feasible with formalin-fixed paraffin-embedded (FFPE) tissue.

2. Applications:
   - Simultaneous evaluation of:
     - MYCN amplification.
     - Segmental Chromosomal Aberrations (SCAs).
     - ALK alterations.
3. Recommended Panel/Approach:
   - Robust assessment of copy number status.
   - Adequate coverage of:
     - ALK regions.
     - Other neuroblastoma-associated genes.

Other Methods

1. FISH and Microarray:
   - Can evaluate standard prognostic biomarkers (e.g., MYCN, SCAs).
   - Limitations:
   - Do not identify sequence variants in ALK or other neuroblastoma-associated genes.

Germline Alterations

1. Incidental Findings:
   - Genetic alterations related to cancer predisposition or inherited conditions may be identified during:
     - Single-gene testing.
     - Broad testing approaches.
2. Indications for Dedicated Germline Testing:
   - Based on:
     - Family history.
     - Clinical presentation.

- Alterations found during molecular tumor profiling.
3. Genetic Counseling:
   - Involvement of:
     - Genetic counselors.
     - Molecular laboratory professionals experienced in germline genetics.
   - Role:
   - Distinguish between germline and somatic variants.
   - Support patients and families in understanding and navigating these findings.

SURGERY: AN IN-DEPTH EXPLORATION

Surgery plays a pivotal role in the treatment of neuroblastoma, but its timing and extent depend on the patient's risk classification, the tumor's characteristics, and the presence of image-defined risk factors (IDRFs). Multidisciplinary collaboration is essential to ensure the best outcomes while minimizing complications.

Pre-Surgical Evaluation

- Imaging for Resectability: Cross-sectional imaging using CT or MRI is critical for assessing the resectability of the primary tumor and identifying IDRFs, which indicate potential surgical risks.
- Multidisciplinary Discussion: Decisions about the risks, benefits, and timing of surgery (upfront or post-neoadjuvant chemotherapy) must involve a team including surgeons, radiologists, oncologists, radiation oncologists, and pathologists.

General Surgical Principles

Understanding the heterogeneous behavior of neuroblastoma is vital to determining the appropriate surgical approach:
- Intermediate-Risk Disease: These patients often require a combination of surgery and

chemotherapy. When significant surgical risks exist, neoadjuvant chemotherapy should precede surgery to reduce tumor size and surgical complications.

- High-Risk Disease: Neoadjuvant chemotherapy is almost always indicated before attempting resection to reduce tumor burden and facilitate safer surgery.
- Conservative Approach: For all risk groups, surgery should aim to:
  - Minimize morbidity and mortality.
  - Avoid resecting vital structures unnecessarily.
  - Preserve organ function wherever possible.

Principles of Tumor Biopsy

When upfront tumor resection is not feasible or recommended due to clinical considerations, a biopsy should be performed to enable diagnosis and risk stratification:
- Indications:
  - Patients with metastatic disease.
  - Patients with L2 tumors, characterized by the presence of IDRFs and more complex surgical risks.
- Biopsy Techniques:
  - Incisional Biopsy: Performed through an open or laparoscopic/thoracoscopic approach. It should collect at least 1 cm^3 of fresh viable tissue for diagnostic and risk stratification purposes.
  - Core Biopsy: Can be done by a surgeon or interventional radiologist, collecting at least 10

cores of adequate tissue to allow comprehensive analysis.
- Pathologist Assessment: Immediate evaluation of the biopsy by a pathologist is crucial to confirm that the tissue is viable and diagnostic rather than necrotic.

Surgical Approach by Risk Group in Neuroblastoma

The surgical management of neuroblastoma varies significantly based on the risk classification of the disease and specific patient characteristics. Key principles for each risk group are outlined below.

Low-Risk Neuroblastoma

- Primary Role of Surgery: Patients with INRG Stage L1 tumors are often cured with surgical resection. If upfront surgery can be performed safely and potentially eliminate the need for chemotherapy, it should be pursued.
- Observation in Specific Cases: For infants where observation without biopsy or resection is deemed appropriate, surgery may not be necessary. This is particularly relevant in certain cases of small, localized tumors.

Intermediate-Risk Neuroblastoma

- Role of IDRFs: The decision to perform upfront resection without chemotherapy depends on the absence or presence of IDRFs (L1 vs. L2 disease) and

the risk of surgical morbidity as assessed by the surgeon.
- Neoadjuvant Chemotherapy: If IDRFs are present or the risk of surgical morbidity is significant, neoadjuvant chemotherapy is recommended to reduce the tumor size and improve the safety of resection.
- Surgical Goals:
  - Attempt gross total resection after systemic therapy when possible. However, achieving less than a complete response is acceptable as long as vital structures and organ function are preserved.
  - The timing of surgery should be based on the tumor's response to initial therapy and ongoing assessments of surgical risk.

High-Risk Neuroblastoma

- Timing of Surgery: Surgery is typically performed before completing Induction therapy, as extending preoperative chemotherapy beyond multiple cycles is unlikely to further reduce surgical risks.
- Surgical Goals:
  - Attempt maximal safe resection of the primary tumor, but avoid removing residual disease adherent to vital structures to prevent significant morbidity or delays in postoperative systemic therapy.
  - Organ Preservation: Do not remove adjacent organs such as the kidney, pancreas, or intestine unless absolutely necessary. These resections can increase surgical complications and negatively

affect subsequent therapies. Nephrectomy is specifically discouraged due to the potential for renal toxicity from neuroblastoma treatments.

- Vascular Encasement: Tumors encasing major blood vessels require careful identification, isolation, and dissection. Avoid dissecting deeper than the adventitial layer to minimize the risk of vascular injury. Tumors can be removed in segments; en bloc resection is not mandatory.

- Nodal Disease: Resection of nodal disease adherent to the primary tumor is encouraged, provided it does not increase morbidity. However, resection of distant lymph nodes during primary tumor surgery is not required.

Special Considerations for Infants with INRG MS Disease

- Primary Surgical Role: In cases of MS disease, the surgical goal is to obtain tissue for histologic and biologic analysis through a biopsy of the primary or metastatic tumor when safe.
- Risk of Surgical Complications: Infants under 3 months with massive hepatomegaly or coagulopathy are at higher risk of complications. In such cases, systemic therapy may precede biopsy. Biopsy can be delayed until conditions improve and surgery becomes safe.
- Severe Hepatomegaly with Respiratory Compromise: In extreme cases where respiratory distress or life-threatening symptoms occur,

laparotomy with silo placement may be performed to relieve intra-abdominal pressure.

Surgical Management of Cervical and Cervicothoracic Neuroblastoma

Preoperative Assessments:

- Evaluate tumor involvement with critical structures, including the vertebral and carotid arteries, jugular vein, subclavian vessels, brachial plexus roots, and extension across the midline or to the base of the skull.
- Assess for tracheal compression using patient symptoms or cross-sectional imaging before proceeding with general anesthesia.
- If the tumor extends into the thoracic cavity, consider advanced surgical approaches such as a cervicothoracic "trap door" incision or median sternotomy with cervical extension for effective access.

Intraoperative Considerations:

- Preserve critical nerves such as the vagus nerve, brachial plexus, phrenic nerve, and others. Use intraoperative nerve monitoring to enhance safety during dissection.
- Coordinate with the anesthesia team regarding neuromuscular blockade, as it may interfere with nerve monitoring.

- Postoperative Horner's Syndrome: Inform families about the possibility of this complication, which may occur after resections involving neck and apical chest tumors.

Lymphadenectomy:

- Complete compartment-oriented cervical lymphadenectomy is not recommended in these cases.

Surgical Management of Thoracic Cavity Neuroblastoma

Preoperative Assessments:

- Evaluate for tumor encasement of critical structures such as the thoracic aorta, vena cava, and other great vessels.
- Assess for tracheal compression using patient symptoms or imaging before administering general anesthesia.
- Use spine MRI if the tumor involves the spinal foraminae or if symptoms suggest spinal extension.

Surgical Approaches:

- Thoracotomy is preferred for large tumors or those involving critical thoracic structures.
- Thoracoscopy may be suitable for smaller, localized lesions and is the recommended approach for biopsies.

Nerve and Spinal Considerations:

- Avoid aggressive resection, retraction, or monopolar cautery near critical nerves such as the recurrent laryngeal, phrenic, and vagus nerves.
- Minimize risk to spinal nerve roots by avoiding deep or blind tissue dissection in regions of neural foraminal extension. Residual tumor in these areas may be left to prevent neurologic injury.
- For cases with known intraspinal extension, involve the multidisciplinary team, often including neurosurgery.

Spinal Cord and Vascular Preservation:

- Preoperatively evaluate thoracic imaging for arterial branches to the spinal cord, including the artery of Adamkiewicz. Preserve these vessels, especially for tumors involving multiple thoracic levels, even if leaving residual tumor is necessary.

Thoracic Duct Management:

- Dissect carefully near the carina and right hemidiaphragm to prevent injury to the thoracic duct.
- Seal or ligate any visible lymphatic structures and inspect thoroughly for leaks before completing the procedure.

Surgical Management for Neuroblastoma in Abdominal, Adrenal, Retroperitoneal, and Pelvic Cavities

Preoperative Assessments and Considerations:

- Critical Vessel Involvement: Evaluate the tumor's relationship to vital structures such as the porta hepatis, hepatoduodenal ligament, mesenteric arteries, celiac axis, aorta, vena cava, and iliac vessels. Surgical resection should avoid compromising these vessels to minimize risks such as bowel ischemia. Proximal and distal vascular control should be established when necessary.
- Renal Structures: Assess for tumor infiltration of renal pedicles and ensure that nephrectomy is avoided unless absolutely unavoidable. Ureteral involvement is possible, requiring meticulous dissection to prevent injury.
- Nerve Involvement: In pelvic tumors, preoperative MRI should evaluate potential involvement of nerve roots and sacral structures, given the proximity to the lumbosacral plexus and obturator nerve. Intraoperative nerve monitoring is recommended.

Surgical Approaches:

- Laparoscopic Surgery: This may be considered depending on the tumor's size, location, and relationship to nearby structures, provided it does not compromise the completeness or safety of resection.
- Tumor Adherence to Critical Structures: If tumors are adherent to vital organs or structures, leaving a small residual tumor may be necessary to avoid major complications.

Surgical Management for Paraspinal Tumors

Preoperative Steps:

- Neurologic Assessment: A comprehensive preoperative neurologic examination should document any existing deficits. This will guide the surgical plan and postoperative monitoring.
- Spinal Imaging: Obtain a preoperative spine MRI to evaluate the tumor's relationship with the spinal cord and nerve roots.

Management of Neurologic Risks:

- In cases with neurologic symptoms or acute spinal cord compression, rapid initiation of chemotherapy is often the first step. Surgical intervention, such as laminectomy, is rarely indicated at diagnosis.
- If progressive neurologic symptoms occur despite systemic therapy, a multidisciplinary re-evaluation should be conducted urgently.

Intraoperative Considerations and Complications

General Intraoperative Challenges:
1. Hemorrhage:
   - Hemorrhage is a significant risk, especially with infiltrative tumors involving major vessels.
   - Preoperative planning should involve potential consultation with vascular surgeons. If critical vessels such as the aorta, carotid, subclavian,

or renal arteries are injured, repair should be performed either primarily or using a graft to restore blood flow.

2. Nerve Injury:

- The risk of nerve injury varies by tumor site. If nerves are damaged, intraoperative consultation with neurosurgery or plastic surgery specialists is advised for possible repair.

Decision-Making in Tumor Resection

- Leaving residual tumor that is adherent to vital structures is an acceptable and recommended strategy when aggressive resection poses a significant risk of injury to critical vessels or nerves. Document the extent of tumor resection clearly in the operative report for accurate postoperative planning.

SYSTEMIC THERAPY: AN IN-DEPTH EXPLORATION

Systemic therapy in neuroblastoma, particularly for low- and intermediate-risk patients, aims to achieve excellent survival outcomes while minimizing treatment intensity for those with favorable disease biology. Recent clinical trials have successfully demonstrated that therapy reduction in patients with favorable tumor features can maintain high survival rates, ensuring a balance between efficacy and minimized toxicity.

Over the last two decades, neuroblastoma management has undergone significant advancements, including the evolution of staging systems, risk classification criteria, and response assessments. Historically, clinical trials utilized the legacy International Neuroblastoma Staging System (INSS) and earlier response evaluation methods. The latest guidelines now incorporate data from these trials while aligning with current staging systems, such as the International Neuroblastoma Risk Group Staging System (INRGSS) and modern response criteria. However, legacy methods remain relevant in certain contexts.

Low-Risk Neuroblastoma

For patients with INRG Stage L1 tumors, surgical resection is the primary treatment, except in specific cases:

- Infants under 6 months of age with adrenal tumors ≤3.1 cm in diameter (solid) or ≤5 cm (with at least 25% cystic components) are candidates for observation without biopsy.
- Asymptomatic patients with INRG Stage MS disease and favorable tumor biology are also managed with observation alone.

Intermediate-Risk Neuroblastoma

Patients with intermediate-risk disease undergo moderate-intensity multi-agent chemotherapy combined with surgical resection. The COG ANBL0531 trial refined treatment strategies by reducing the number of chemotherapy cycles for patients with favorable biology, allowing for greater residual tumor volume post-treatment compared to prior protocols. Key features of the approach include:

- The number of chemotherapy cycles is determined by patient age, tumor stage, and biologic characteristics.
- After completing the prescribed cycles, disease response is assessed to guide decisions on further therapy, surgery, or surveillance.

The ANBL0531 trial set specific response targets:

- For localized tumors with favorable biology, the goal was a 50% reduction in tumor volume.
- For less favorable localized disease, therapy continued until a 90% reduction in tumor volume (very good partial response [VGPR]).
- For metastatic disease (e.g., INRG MS or M stage disease), response goals were trial-specific and did not align with legacy criteria.

Since the trial's completion, response criteria have shifted from tumor volume measurements to single-dimensional assessments using the RECIST criteria (Response Evaluation Criteria in Solid Tumors). While VGPR is no longer a recognized category, current recommendations permit using either volume or single-dimension measurements for evaluating responses in non-high-risk patients until additional data emerge.

Addressing Incomplete Responses

When the targeted tumor reduction is not achieved with the initial chemotherapy regimen, multidisciplinary discussions are essential to determine the next steps. Options include:

- Surgical Resection: If deemed safe and feasible, surgery may achieve the desired response endpoint.
- Additional Chemotherapy: For patients where surgery is too risky, additional chemotherapy cycles are administered with reevaluation after every two cycles.
- Biopsy of Residual Mass: In certain cases, biopsy

may assess histologic differentiation to support observation of stable residual tumors where surgical debulking is unsafe.

The ANBL0531 trial identified cyclophosphamide and topotecan as effective additional treatments for intermediate-risk patients who did not meet response targets after the initial eight cycles of therapy. Similar outcomes have been achieved using SIOPEN (European-based) regimens, providing alternative treatment pathways.

High-Risk Neuroblastoma: Induction Therapy

Patients newly diagnosed with high-risk neuroblastoma face significant challenges, with an estimated 5-year event-free survival (EFS) rate of 51%, based on a decade of data from the Children's Oncology Group (COG). Despite these odds, survival outcomes have steadily improved through the development of intensive multimodal therapies, which are divided into three phases: Induction, Consolidation, and Post-Consolidation. Participation in clinical trials is highly encouraged whenever available, as they continue to shape advancements in treatment strategies.

Goals of Induction Therapy

The primary objective of Induction therapy is to reduce the tumor burden and achieve the best possible response before advancing to the next

phases of treatment. This phase typically involves:
- Multiagent Chemotherapy: Administered to aggressively target the cancer cells.
- Surgical Resection: To remove as much of the primary tumor as safely possible.
- Stem Cell Collection: Autologous peripheral blood stem cells are harvested during Induction for use in subsequent therapy phases, particularly in high-dose chemotherapy with stem cell rescue.

Evolution of Induction Regimens

Over the last two decades, various Induction chemotherapy regimens have been developed and tested in North American cooperative group trials and pilot studies. These regimens generally aim to balance treatment efficacy with minimizing toxicity. Although no randomized trials directly compare the effectiveness of these regimens, they have shown broadly similar outcomes, achieving:
- Approximately 80% partial response (PR) or better by the end of Induction.
- About 9% disease progression despite aggressive treatment.

Toxicity concerns have driven changes to reduce the use of nephrotoxic (kidney-damaging) and cardiotoxic (heart-damaging) agents, ensuring safer but still effective treatment strategies.

Key Trials and Regimens

- Topotecan and Cyclophosphamide Regimen: Early studies demonstrated an 84% end-Induction response rate using these agents in the initial cycles of therapy. This regimen was adopted in the ANBL0532 trial, where 39.1% of patients achieved PR or better after just two cycles.

- Five-Cycle Regimens: The ANBL12P1 trial reduced the number of Induction cycles to five, achieving an 80% end-Induction response rate. Comparable outcomes were observed with 5-cycle versus 7-cycle regimens in data from Memorial Sloan-Kettering Cancer Center (MSKCC).

- Standard Regimens: The ANBL1531 trial adopted a 5-cycle Induction regimen similar to ANBL12P1, with minor adjustments to dosing for alignment with updated COG chemotherapy standards.

Recommendations

- Preferred Regimens: ANBL12P1 or ANBL1531, which both employ 5 cycles of Induction therapy.
- Alternative Regimen: A 6-cycle regimen from ANBL0532, though less commonly used, is an acceptable option.
- Flexibility: Other published regimens with similar response rates may also be appropriate for individual patients based on specific clinical considerations.

While the lack of comparative data among regimens limits direct recommendations, these therapies provide a robust framework for achieving strong responses during the Induction phase. This foundational treatment sets the stage for advancing to Consolidation and Post-Consolidation therapies, which further aim to maximize survival outcomes in high-risk neuroblastoma.

Enhancements and Considerations in Induction Therapy for High-Risk Neuroblastoma

Efforts are ongoing to improve Induction therapy for high-risk neuroblastoma, targeting better outcomes and reducing treatment-related risks. While these strategies remain under investigation, they highlight the evolving approach to this aggressive disease.

Emerging Strategies

Several promising interventions are being evaluated, including:

- ALK Inhibitors: For patients with tumors harboring ALK aberrations, early addition of an ALK inhibitor is under study.

- 131I-MIBG Therapy: Early administration of this radiopharmaceutical, which targets neuroblastoma cells, is being explored.

- Anti-GD2 Monoclonal Antibody Therapy: Investigations are focusing on its early use during Induction.

While these approaches show potential, the guidelines do not recommend their routine use outside of clinical trials until robust safety and efficacy data are available.

Surgical Goals in Induction

Surgical resection of the primary tumor and nearby lymph nodes is a key goal during Induction therapy. However, due to the aggressive nature of high-risk neuroblastoma, upfront surgery is rarely feasible. Instead, the guidelines recommend surgical intervention after several cycles of cytoreductive chemotherapy to reduce tumor size and minimize surgical risks.

- Extent of Resection: Complete microscopic resection is rarely achievable or recommended due to the risk of damaging vital structures such as organs, nerves, or blood vessels. Instead, the goal is gross total resection, which entails removing >90% of the tumor.

- Subtotal Resection: When vital structures are at risk, a subtotal resection is advised to prioritize patient safety.

Studies from North America and Europe support the benefits of achieving gross total resection, showing improved event-free survival (EFS) and reduced rates of local relapse or progression.

End-Induction Reassessment

A full disease evaluation at the end of Induction is a pivotal step in treatment. This evaluation helps determine the next phase of therapy and assesses patient response:

- Response Categories:

- Patients with a partial response or better typically proceed to Consolidation therapy.
- Those with progressive disease are not candidates for Consolidation and instead receive non-myeloablative therapies, such as chemoimmunotherapy with anti-GD2 monoclonal antibodies or enrollment in clinical trials.
- Patients with minor response or stable disease require individualized treatment planning, including consideration of bridging therapies.

Role of Bridging Therapy

For patients with incomplete response to Induction, bridging therapies aim to improve outcomes before advancing to Consolidation. Retrospective data suggest that:
- Patients achieving a complete response with bridging therapy and proceeding to Consolidation therapy show favorable outcomes.
- Even those with partial improvement from bridging therapies benefit more from Consolidation than those who stop after bridging.

Consolidation Therapy for High-Risk Neuroblastoma

Consolidation therapy is a critical phase in the treatment of high-risk neuroblastoma, aiming to eliminate residual disease after Induction therapy. It typically involves high-dose chemotherapy with autologous stem cell rescue (HSCT) and radiotherapy to the primary tumor site. In North America, radiotherapy to residual metastatic disease sites identified at the end of Induction is also considered standard practice.

High-Dose Chemotherapy with Autologous Stem Cell Rescue

- Proven Benefits: This approach has been foundational in high-risk neuroblastoma treatment, with randomized trials showing improved survival compared to continued conventional chemotherapy. However, these studies were conducted before the routine use of anti-GD2 immunotherapy, raising questions about the necessity of HSCT in certain subgroups in the modern era.

- Tandem Transplantation: For most high-risk patients, the guidelines recommend two consecutive rounds of high-dose chemotherapy with autologous stem cell rescue (tandem transplantation). Evidence from the COG ANBL0532 trial demonstrated superior 3-year event-free survival (EFS) rates for tandem transplantation (61.6%) compared to a single transplant (48.4%).

- Single Transplant Subgroups: A single round of HSCT may be appropriate for patients with:

1. Stage L2 disease, age ≥18 months, unfavorable histology, and MYCN non-amplified disease.

2. Stage M disease, age 12 to <18 months, MYCN non-amplified, with one or more unfavorable features (unfavorable histology, diploid DNA

content, or segmental chromosomal aberrations).

These patients historically have more favorable outcomes, with 5-year EFS rates of 75%–80%. For such cases, single transplantation with carboplatin/etoposide/melphalan (CEM) is endorsed.

Conditioning Regimens

- Busulfan and Melphalan (BuMel): This regimen is preferred in Europe, where a randomized phase 3 trial showed superior EFS with BuMel compared to CEM following rapid COJEC Induction. BuMel was also associated with fewer adverse events overall, although it increased the risk of sinusoidal obstruction syndrome. The COG ANBL12P1 trial demonstrated the feasibility of BuMel in North America, but its role in this context is not yet fully established. BuMel may be suitable for patients with contraindications to tandem transplantation or those eligible for single transplantation.

Radiotherapy

- Primary Tumor Site: Radiotherapy is typically administered after recovery from HSCT. Neuroblastoma is highly radiosensitive, and a dose of 21.6 Gy is commonly used.
- Residual Metastatic Disease: Radiation to metastatic sites remaining at the end of Induction is recommended, although not all sites can be feasibly targeted. Single-institution studies support the efficacy of this approach, but it has not been universally adopted.

- Augmented Doses: Trials such as COG A3973 and ANBL0532 evaluated extending radiotherapy to uninvolved nodal stations or boosting doses to gross residual tumors. Neither approach showed additional benefits in reducing local relapse or improving EFS and is not recommended.

Considerations for Future Studies

While current standards emphasize the combination of high-dose chemotherapy, HSCT, and radiotherapy, the emergence of anti-GD2 immunotherapy highlights the need for further research to optimize Consolidation therapy. Identifying subgroups that may benefit from less intensive approaches remains a priority to balance efficacy and toxicity.

Post-Consolidation Therapy for High-Risk Neuroblastoma

Post-consolidation therapy is a vital phase in high-risk neuroblastoma treatment, aimed at further reducing the risk of relapse after induction and consolidation. Its strategies have evolved over time, incorporating new therapies and evidence-based practices.

Historical and Current Approaches

- Isotretinoin Therapy: Historically, six cycles of isotretinoin were used as a differentiating agent in post-consolidation therapy. This approach was supported by the CCG-3891 trial, which showed improved outcomes with isotretinoin compared to no additional therapy.

- Anti-GD2 Monoclonal Antibody Therapy: The ANBL0032 trial demonstrated a significant improvement in event-free survival (EFS) when combining dinutuximab, cytokines (sargramostim and interleukin-2), and isotretinoin compared to isotretinoin alone. This regimen achieved a 2-year EFS of 66%, compared to 46% with isotretinoin alone, establishing it as the standard post-consolidation therapy.

Refinements in Anti-GD2 Therapy

- Recent data from the SIOPEN HR-NBL1 trial questioned the role of interleukin-2 in combination with anti-GD2 immunotherapy, finding no improvement in outcomes and increased toxicity. Based on these findings, interleukin-2 is no longer included in COG protocols.
- Alternative anti-GD2 regimens, such as dinutuximab beta with isotretinoin but without sargramostim, are commonly used in Europe. These regimens have shown higher EFS rates compared to isotretinoin alone in non-randomized comparisons.

Continuation Therapy

Continuation therapy using eflornithine (DFMO), an inhibitor of polyamine synthesis, has emerged as a promising addition for patients with high-risk neuroblastoma who respond to frontline therapy.

- Clinical Trial Evidence: In a Phase 2 trial (Study 3b), children receiving eflornithine after induction, consolidation, and anti-GD2 immunotherapy demonstrated significantly better outcomes than a control group that did not receive continuation therapy. The trial reported:
  - EFS hazard ratio: 0.48 (95% CI: 0.27–0.85).
  - Overall survival (OS) hazard ratio: 0.32 (95% CI: 0.15–0.70).
- FDA Approval: Based on these findings, the FDA approved eflornithine in December 2023 for use in continuation therapy for high-risk neuroblastoma patients achieving a partial response or better after anti-GD2 immunotherapy.
- Adverse Effects: Reported side effects include transaminitis and hearing loss, necessitating regular monitoring.
- Recommendations: Clinicians are encouraged to discuss eflornithine as a therapy option with families.

Disease Evaluations During Therapy

Frequent and comprehensive disease evaluations are essential throughout frontline therapy to guide treatment adjustments and assess response:
- Staging Evaluations: Anatomic imaging (CT or MRI) of the primary tumor site is performed prior to planned surgical resection.

- End-Induction and Post-Consolidation Evaluations:
  - Full disease assessments, including 123I-MIBG scans (or FDG-PET for MIBG non-avid tumors) and bone marrow biopsies, are conducted at key milestones: the end of induction, start of post-consolidation therapy, and end of therapy.
  - For patients with more than five MIBG-avid metastatic sites at the end of induction, repeat scans are recommended after recovery from high-dose chemotherapy to prioritize metastatic sites for consolidative radiotherapy.
- Mid-Therapy Evaluations: During post-consolidation therapy, a repeat MIBG or FDG-PET scan is performed halfway through treatment, with additional imaging reserved for patients with residual disease.

Organ Function Monitoring

High-risk neuroblastoma therapy is intensive and associated with both acute and long-term toxicities, requiring vigilant monitoring:
- Renal Function: Assessed through nuclear medicine tests of glomerular filtration rate before high-dose chemotherapy.
- Cardiac Function: Serial evaluations using electrocardiograms and echocardiograms.
- Hearing: Regular audiograms or brainstem auditory evoked response tests are crucial, as most patients are at a critical age for language development.

Therapy for Adolescents and Adults

Although neuroblastoma is predominantly a pediatric disease, adolescents and adults may occasionally present with high-risk cases. For these patients:

- The same general treatment principles apply.
- However, therapy must be individualized based on comorbid conditions and tolerance to the intensive regimens, given the limited data for older populations.

RADIATION THERAPY: AN IN-DEPTH EXPLORATION

Radiation therapy (RT) is **a critical component of treatment for high-risk neuroblastoma and is typically not used for patients with non–high-risk disease**. Its application follows recovery from high-dose chemotherapy with stem cell rescue unless there is an urgent need for RT.

General Principles

- Timing: RT is administered after recovery from high-dose chemotherapy unless emergent indications require earlier intervention.
- Techniques: Intensity-modulated radiation therapy (IMRT) or proton therapy is preferred to minimize side effects and reduce radiation exposure to healthy tissues.
- Targets:
  - The primary tumor site is always irradiated.
  - Metastatic sites are treated if there is evidence of active disease, such as MIBG/FDG uptake or a persistent soft-tissue mass greater than 1 cm^3 after induction chemotherapy.
  - Metastatic and primary sites should be irradiated concurrently when indicated.
- Feasibility: Not all metastatic sites may be practically targeted with external beam RT. Recommendations to irradiate metastatic sites are

supported by single-institution data but have not been universally adopted.

Simulation

- Patients are positioned supine with proper immobilization for CT simulation.
- For targets influenced by respiratory motion, 4D-CT is recommended.
- MRI simulation may be considered for paraspinal tumor sites to enhance precision.

Target Volume Definitions

1. Primary Site:
   - Gross Tumor Volume (GTV): Includes the postoperative tumor bed, any residual disease, and initially involved regional lymph nodes. Defined using post-induction chemotherapy imaging fused with pre-surgical imaging studies.
   - Special consideration: For tumors resected before induction chemotherapy, GTV is based on the initial tumor volume at diagnosis.
   - Clinical Target Volume (CTV): Defined as GTV plus 1 cm but confined to anatomical borders, avoiding uninvolved organs like kidneys, bones, or abdominal structures.
   - Internal Target Volume (ITV): Accounts for respiratory motion when necessary, based on 4D-CT.
   - Planning Target Volume (PTV): Combines CTV with an additional 0.3–0.5 cm, adjusted per institutional standards and immobilization

methods.

2. Metastatic Sites:
- Metastatic GTV (mGTV): Defined by post-induction chemotherapy imaging.
- Metastatic CTV (mCTV): mGTV plus 1 cm, confined to anatomical borders.
- Metastatic PTV (mPTV): mCTV plus 0.3–0.5 cm, depending on institutional practices.
- Special Consideration: For brain metastases, treatment of the entire craniospinal axis may be considered due to the high risk of distant central nervous system (CNS) relapse.

Radiation Dose

- Neuroblastoma is highly radiosensitive. A standard dose of 21.6 Gy is recommended for local control.
- Augmented radiation doses have not shown significant improvements in local disease control in recent trials.

Response Assessment

The International Neuroblastoma Response Criteria (INRC) serve as the standardized framework for assessing tumor response during and after treatment. It incorporates evaluations of the primary tumor site, metastatic lesions, and bone marrow involvement using modern imaging and functional assessment tools.

PRIMARY TUMOR RESPONSE ASSESSMENT: AN IN-DEPTH EXPLORATION

Methodology

- RECIST (Response Evaluation Criteria in Solid Tumors) guidelines are used for soft-tissue measurements.
- Functional imaging, such as MIBG scintigraphy or FDG-PET (for MIBG non-avid tumors), is incorporated to evaluate metabolic activity.

Criteria for Response

1. Complete Response (CR):
   - Residual soft tissue at the primary site measures less than 10 mm.
   - Complete resolution of MIBG or FDG-PET uptake at the primary site.

2. Partial Response (PR):
   - At least a 30% reduction in the longest diameter of the primary tumor.
   - MIBG or FDG-PET uptake at the primary site is stable, improved, or resolved.

3. Stable Disease (SD):
   - Neither sufficient shrinkage to qualify as PR nor

sufficient growth to classify as progressive disease (PD) is observed.

4. Progressive Disease (PD):

- Tumor size increases by more than 20% in the longest diameter, taking the smallest recorded diameter as a reference (including the baseline measurement if it is the smallest observed).

- The absolute increase in the longest dimension must be at least 5 mm.

Response Assessment for Metastatic Bone and Soft Tissue Lesions in Neuroblastoma

The International Neuroblastoma Response Criteria (INRC) provides a systematic framework for assessing the response of metastatic bone and soft tissue lesions during and after treatment. The criteria utilize a combination of RECIST measurements, modified Curie or SIOPEN scores, and functional imaging (MIBG or FDG-PET) to evaluate disease status.

Criteria for Response

1. Complete Response (CR):

- All non-primary target lesions and non-target lesions are reduced to <10 mm in size.

- Lymph nodes that were identified as target lesions decrease to a short axis of <10 mm.

- MIBG uptake or FDG-PET uptake in non-primary

lesions resolves completely.

2. Partial Response (PR):
   - At least a 30% decrease in the sum of diameters of non-primary target lesions compared to baseline.
   - All of the following must also be true:
     - Non-target lesions are stable or smaller.
     - No new lesions are detected.
   - A ≥50% reduction in the absolute MIBG bone score (relative score between 0.1 and 0.5) or in the number of FDG-PET avid bone lesions.

3. Stable Disease (SD):
   - Changes in non-primary lesions do not meet the criteria for PR or PD (progressive disease).

4. Progressive Disease (PD):
   - Any of the following indicates progression:
     - New soft tissue lesions detected by CT/MRI that are also MIBG avid or FDG-PET avid.
     - New soft tissue lesions on anatomic imaging that are biopsied and confirmed to be neuroblastoma or ganglioneuroblastoma.
     - Any new MIBG-avid bone site.
     - New FDG-PET avid bone site (for MIBG non-avid tumors) confirmed by CT/MRI or biopsy.
   - More than 20% increase in the sum of the longest diameters of target soft tissue lesions, with an absolute increase of at least 5 mm.
   - A relative MIBG bone score of ≥1.2.

Response Assessment for Bone

Marrow in Neuroblastoma

The International Neuroblastoma Response Criteria (INRC), supported by Burchill et al., provides detailed guidelines for assessing bone marrow response to treatment. This involves evaluating the level of tumor infiltration in the bone marrow during and after therapy.

Bone Marrow Response Criteria

1. Complete Response (CR):
 - No tumor infiltration is detected in the bone marrow upon reassessment, regardless of the level of infiltration at baseline.

2. Minimal Disease (MD):
 - Bone marrow infiltration meets one of the following criteria:
    - Tumor infiltration is reduced to ≤5% but remains above 0%.
    - No tumor infiltration is detected initially, but reassessment shows infiltration of ≤5%.
    - Initial infiltration of >20% is reduced to >0% to ≤5% upon reassessment.

3. Stable Disease (SD):
 - Tumor infiltration remains positive and exceeds 5%, without meeting the thresholds for CR, MD, or PD.

4. Progressive Disease (PD):
 - Bone marrow without prior tumor infiltration

shows >5% tumor infiltration upon reassessment.

- Tumor infiltration in the bone marrow increases by more than 2-fold, and the level exceeds 20% upon reassessment.

Overall Response Assessment for Neuroblastoma

The International Neuroblastoma Response Criteria (INRC) aggregates the response evaluations of various components (primary tumor, metastatic sites, bone marrow, etc.) to determine the overall treatment response. The classification ensures a comprehensive view of the disease status based on the best and worst outcomes across all components.

Overall Response Categories

1. Complete Response (CR):
   - Achieved when all components meet the criteria for complete response (CR) with no evidence of residual disease.

2. Progressive Disease (PD):
   - Defined when any single component meets the criteria for progressive disease (PD), regardless of the status of other components.

3. Partial Response (PR):
   - Achieved when at least one component shows partial response (PR) and all other components show one of the following:
     - Complete response (CR).

- Minimal disease (MD) (bone marrow).
- Partial response (PR).
- No involvement at baseline.

4. Minor Response (MR):

- Defined when at least one component shows partial response (PR) or complete response (CR), but at least one other component shows stable disease (SD).

- No component should meet the criteria for progressive disease (PD).

5. Stable Disease (SD):

- Occurs when at least one component shows stable disease (SD), and no other component demonstrates a response better than stable disease or was uninvolved at baseline.

A LETTER TO FAMILIES

Dearest reader,

You are now confronted with a challenge of considerable magnitude—neuroblastoma. This is no trivial matter, but neither is it one devoid of hope or opportunity. It is critical, as you face this challenge, to fortify yourselves with knowledge, resilience, and a commitment to action, for the stakes are high, and the pathway forward demands nothing less than your full engagement.

Neuroblastoma arises from immature nerve cells in the sympathetic nervous system, typically presenting in young children. Its clinical presentation varies widely—some cases are highly treatable, while others require the full arsenal of modern medicine. Tumors often originate in the adrenal glands or along the spine and may spread to bones, bone marrow, or lymph nodes. This diversity of presentation means treatment must be tailored to the individual, with interventions that can include surgery, chemotherapy, radiation, immunotherapy, and stem cell transplantation.

These treatments are not without cost. Chemotherapy, for example, is a powerful tool, but it can damage not only the tumor but healthy tissue, leading to side effects such as anemia, immunosuppression, and even organ toxicity. Radiation can precisely target disease but risks damaging surrounding structures. Immunotherapy, particularly anti-GD2 monoclonal antibodies, represents a leap forward in targeted treatment, yet the intense pain during infusions is a stark reminder of the complexity of these approaches.

It is critical to acknowledge the stakes: approximately half of high-risk neuroblastoma cases lead to relapse despite aggressive treatment. Yet this does not mean the fight is lost; it means the battle requires strategy, persistence, and adaptability. It is essential to remember that survival rates have improved, thanks to scientific advances and relentless clinical effort.

Now, what does this mean for you? First, it means a radical acceptance of the situation. This is not to be confused with resignation, but with a determined willingness to confront the problem head-on. Every treatment decision, every test, every adjustment to therapy becomes a step in this process. You must position yourselves as partners with the medical team, fully informed, actively participating, and relentlessly advocating for the best possible care.

Second, recognize that your presence as family is pivotal. You provide not just logistical support but the emotional foundation on which your child will build their resilience. Studies have repeatedly demonstrated the importance of psychological well-being in medical outcomes. Be attentive to your child's needs and your own. Self-care is not a luxury—it is a necessity.

Finally, arm yourselves with knowledge. Seek to understand the mechanisms of the disease and the rationale behind each treatment. This isn't simply to satisfy curiosity; it's to transform fear into competence. When you know why a particular therapy is chosen and what outcomes are expected, you become a more effective advocate.

Let me assure you: this is no journey for the faint of heart, but it is one you are equipped to navigate. Gather your resolve, lean on the community around you, and pursue the best possible outcome with the full force of your capacities. Your child will see your strength and take heart from it.

Every decision you make now contributes to the larger narrative of survival and healing. It is a story of hardship, yes, but also of courage, growth, and —above all—hope. Remember, the darkest chapters are not the end but the turning points, and it is your duty to ensure that this chapter concludes with triumph.

With determination and faith in your capacities,
Dr. Bhratri Bhushan, MD, DM

ABOUT THE AUTHOR

Dr. Bhratri Bhushan

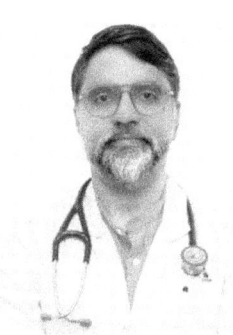

Dr. Bhratri Bhushan is a consultant medical oncologist and hematologist. He has a rich academic and research background, having published more than two hundred books on the subjects of oncology and internal medicine. His scholarly contributions have been featured in renowned journals of medical literature. For a comprehensive collection of his works, please visit his AuthorCentral page at www.amazon.com/author/bhratribhushan

www.ingramcontent.com/pod-product-compliance
Lightning Source LLC
Chambersburg PA
CBHW070145230526
45471CB00002B/527